COMPETITIVE STRATEGY *for*

HEALTH CARE
ORGANIZATIONS

COMPETITIVE STRATEGY *for*

HEALTH CARE
ORGANIZATIONS

TECHNIQUES FOR STRATEGIC ACTION

ALAN SHELDON *and* SUSAN WINDHAM

BeardBooks
Washington, D.C.

Library of Congress Cataloging-in-Publication Data

Sheldon, Alan, 1933-
   Competitive strategy for health care organizations / Alan Sheldon, with Susan Windham.
      p. cm.
   Originally published: Homewood, Ill. : Dow Jones-Irwin, c1984.
   Includes bibliographical references and index.
   ISBN 1-58798-135-1
   1. Medical care--Marketing. 2. Health services administration. 3. Business planning. 4.
Competition. I. Windham, Susan. II. Title

RA410.5 .S65 2002
362.1'068--dc21

                                                    2002028225

Printed in the United States of America

For Pam

PREFACE

In the last 15 years, the environment in which medicine is practiced in the United States has been marked by tumultuous changes. These changes manifest themselves everywhere in the environment: consumer expectations, the flow of funds to providers from public and private third-party payors, capital financing, medical technology, the regulatory environment, and most notably medical costs. At no other time in the history of modern medicine have the providers of health care services faced such floods and fluxes in the information required of them or which they need, or such scrambling for resources; in other words, such uncertainty and competition.

In this competitive and uncertain environment, management skills are at a premium. Health care delivery organizations—hospitals, ambulatory care centers, HMOs, physicians in private practice as individuals or groups—could once effectively survive simply by repeating what they did successfully the year—or decade—before or reacting to events as they happened. To rely upon reaction today is to be the "latest with the least-est." In other words, the current and future competitive and uncertain environment demands not only the development, for the first time, of explicit organizational strategies (i.e., proactive ones), but competitive strategies that result in effective competitive action.

This book addresses the elements of sound strategic action for health care delivery organizations: how managers can decide what to do and make it happen. It is *not* a book for the health system planner or arm-chair economist, but the senior practicing manager whose organization treats patients and who, at the least, must survive and, at best, be successful. The development and implementation of good *competitive* strategy involves, for example, a profound understanding of change. What may need to be done in today's environment may involve great departure from the past, including major changes in the skills and attitudes of staff, and great tact and patience in bringing about the necessary strategic training. Those who deliver health care services have rarely thought carefully about the "market" they serve and tend to regard it as one undifferentiated whole. To provide services competitively, managers of health care organizations must recognize that they serve certain market segments and must understand the concepts of both "product" and "market" to focus energies effectively. To deal with uncertainty in resources, organizations collaborate to aggregate or enter new markets. However, the economical and efficient use of resources often requires restructuring and refocusing them. This book tells you how to take the critical steps that lead to good strategic action.

You will not find any discussion of formal strategic planning here. There are already many excellent works on this subject.[1] Of more importance, however, is the fact that the process of formal strategic planning does not address in reality how top managers make and implement strategies.[2] The book does, however, borrow from previous works on strategic planning where it is germane. The organization of this book is, therefore, untraditional, as it emphasizes strategic action, not planning.

Chapter 1 reviews the eras of medicine, culminating in the present/future so-called era of "network" medicine. This chapter provides the backdrop against which a case is made for the need to develop competitive strategy, introducing as it does the concepts of resource and information uncertainty. The chapter also initiates the competitive analysis, identifying the general environmental trends which influence competitive forces and introducing the idea of relevant environment as an organization shifts from past to future behavior.

Chapter 2 presents the model for competitive strategy development and the competitive forces which impact an organization's relevant envi-

---

[1]George A. Steiner, *Strategic Planning: What Every Manager Must Know* (New York: The Free Press, 1979), and *Top Management Planning* (London: Collier-Macmillan Ltd., 1969).

[2]James B. Quinn, *Strategies for Change: Logical Incrementalism* (Homewood, Ill.: Richard D. Irwin, 1980).

ronment. As the organization readapts from past to future, it engages in a series of positioning actions needed to readjust its competitive position. The positioning actions, described in detail in the second section of the book, are intended to nudge the organization (like tugs on a tanker) in the direction it will ultimately take—its strategy. Several key competitive strategies are described.

Chapters 3-7 detail the positioning actions, those steps which are both strategy implementation and preparation: scanning the environment and the organization; product-market analysis; collaboration; restructuring; managing the physician. Each is discussed at length.

Finally, Chapter 8 describes the competitive issues faced by each type of health care delivery organization: large and small community and teaching hospitals, hospital groups, "super groups," HMOs, IPAs, group practices, nursing homes, home health agencies, and the for-profits, and some generic competitive issues.

The general principles of competitive strategy as described in this book are applicable to senior managers of any kind of health care delivery organization. The details of how they might be applied and enacted will obviously be different, not only in different kinds of organizations, but within a specific organization as it assesses and begins to understand its individual competitive situation. The book can offer guidance but it cannot replace the ultimate managerial skills—good judgment and good timing. The book refers repeatedly to the real dilemmas of managers drawn from the author's experience of over 20 years of teaching, research and consulting. Of course, many examples are disguised to protect confidentiality.

A personal postscript concludes the book, addressed to you who will read and act. A reminder that the management of medicine involves more than you will find in these words with their deliberately limited focus. It requires humanity as well as intelligence, kindness as well as aggressiveness, understanding of personal human suffering as well as the impersonal demands of economics. It requires you to be efficient humanists.

Acknowledgments

We would, most of all, like to thank those individuals and organizations who have shared their experiences and their wisdom with us over the years. The Department of Health Policy and Management, at Harvard School of Public Health, Chairman Professor F. Mosteller, and the Pew Memorial Trust have provided much appreciated continuing financial support. Katy Morakis, and especially Joy Sheldon did a superb job with the typing. Hillary Hart dedicatedly edited even on vacation. Sue Windham would like to give special thanks to her parents, Frank and Ruth Richards, and to David and Colette for their support and encouragement.

Alan Sheldon

CONTENTS

Marketing and Production. The Physician in Institutional Strategy.

Evolution of the Environment: Uncertainty and the Need for Competitive Strategy

Tell me more, with all the authority and brilliance you can muster, about the socio-economic-political structure of the environment in which you attained to the age of reason. Tell me more.

Harold Pinter

The Three Eras of Medical Care

Individual Medicine—The First Era

From 1900 until 1960, the health care environment in this country remained much the same. It was a relatively simple environment, slowly changing. The practice of medicine was characterized by the solo practitioner, working primarily outside medical institutions, paid directly by persons who could afford his services, and providing some amount of free care to those who could not (Figure 1-1). He, because it was rarely she, practiced medicine in preferred isolation, determining which patients would be seen and what treatments would be given. Governance and regulation were overseen by a medical society of peers; the license to practice the profession, once gained, was rarely withdrawn.

During this era of "individual medicine" there were few varieties of health care institutions: acute care hospitals; a few extended stay hospitals for the chronically ill, tubercular, or mentally ill patients; and occasional nursing

1

Figure 1-1

Pre-1960:   Simple Environment
Slow change

Era—Individual Medicine
Few institutions
Few roles
Objectives—not measured
Reactive
Few kinds of education
Education—one time/profession oriented
Service sectors—independent and separate
No priorities
Planning—none
Skills—administrative/status quo
Integration—refer/consult
Emphasis—sick care

---

homes. High-quality, acute care contrasted sharply with an essentially custodial approach to the delivery of chronic care, and both types of institutions were most often fed by general practitioners. Integration among specialists, and between the specialist and general practitioner, was accomplished through informal referrals or consultations. Public health, being practiced in another set of institutions, made enormous strides during this era.

Careers were straightforward: you were trained and went ahead in your profession through easily identifiable mileposts. Institutions had no particular priorities, no clear-cut, measurable objectives, and little relation one to another. Planning, except in public health, was nonexistent.

Organizational Medicine—The Second Era

The era of "organizational medicine" began in the early 60s (Figure 1-2). As the costs and the technological sophistication of medical care increased, the focus of medical care began to shift from the individual practitioner to traditional health care institutions as well as new organizations of physicians. After 1965, this trend was increased by the introduction of Medicare, Medicaid, and other programs of federal support for health care, which infused massive quantities of dollars into the health sector and dramatically increased the accessibility of medical services to

Figure 1-2

```
1960-1975: Complex Environment
            Cost +
         Regulation +
         Technology +
          Change +
         Resources + +

    Era—Organizational Medicine
      More/larger institutions
           More roles
  Emergence of extramural sector
     Objectives—convenient
            Reactive
      Variety of education
  Education—one time/skill oriented
          No priorities
  Planning—constraining growth
   Skills—management/growth
    Integration—refer/consult
  Emphasis—sick care and prevention
Quality of care determined by physician
```

Table 1-1

Selected Data on U.S. Health Care Expenditures, 1940-1980

Year	Total Amount ($ billion)	Percent of GNP	Per Capita Expenditures	Hospital Care ($ billion)	Physicians' Services ($ billion)	Index of Medical Care Prices	Consumer Price Index
1940	$ 4.0	$4.0	$ 29.62	$ 1.01	$ 0.97	36.8	42.0
1950	12.7	4.5	81.86	3.85	2.75	53.7	72.1
1960	26.9	5.3	146.30	9.09	5.68	79.1	88.7
1965	40.5	5.9	204.68	13.61	8.75	89.5	94.5
1970	71.6	7.3	343.44	27.60	14.29	120.6	116.3
1975	131.5	8.6	566.61	52.10	24.90	163.6	161.2
1980*	217.9	9.2	1,067.06	70.60	42.30	265.9	246.8

*HIAA, *Source Book for Health Insurance Data, 1981-82* (Washington, D.C.: Government Printing Office, 1983).

Source: U.S. Bureau of the Census, *Historical Statistics to 1970* (Washington, D.C.: U.S. Government Printing Office); U.S. Bureau of the Census, *Statistical Abstract* (Washington, D.C.: U.S. Government Printing Office, 1979).

Table 1-2

Insurance and the Net Cost of Hospital Care

	1950	1960	1970	1975	1980
Percentage of hospital costs paid by:					
Private insurance	29.30	52.50	45.60	43.60	36.60
Government	21.10	18.80	37.80	44.50	54.20
Direct consumer spending	49.60	28.70	16.60	11.90	9.10
Percentage of private cost of hospital care paid by:					
Private insurance	37.10	64.70	73.20	78.60	—
Direct consumer spending	62.90	35.30	26.80	21.40	—
Average cost per patient day*	15.62	32.23	81.01	151.53	245.60

All figures exclude hospital costs in federal, long-term, tuberculosis, and psychiatric hospitals.

*HIAA, *Source Book for Health Insurance Data, 1981-82* (Washington, D.C.: Government Printing Office, 1983).

Source: Martin S. Feldstein and Amy Taylor, *The Rapid Rise of Hospital Costs* (Washington, D.C.: Council on Wage and Price Stability, 1977), p. 31.

consumers whose demand for care had been previously constrained by the price of services (see Tables 1-1 and 1-2). Financially supported in part by this new pool of health care dollars, and driven by increased consumer demand for care, many kinds of new medical institutions emerged during the 15-year period from 1960 to 1975. Group practice developed on a wide scale, as did the community health center and the health maintenance organization (HMO). The size of the modal traditional care institution increased, as well.

This was an era of abundance in the environment. Money was readily available for new complex technologies, more equipment, more services, and bigger and better buildings. There was little perceived need for priorities or planning, and traditional, largely unstated, competitive values flourished. As the variety of institutions increased, new roles emerged, as well as new forms of education and new career patterns. Physicians no longer had to choose between solo or hospital-based practice, but could work in a group of physicians, a rehabilitation unit, or a rural or inner-city health center. New professionals, such as allied and auxiliary health personnel came into being. Health care administrators, once restricted to training in hospital administration and choosing a career path leading from a small hospital to a large one, could now obtain any one of a number of degrees and faced a bewildering set of choices and career options.

During the era of organizational medicine, a growing emphasis was placed on management, the value of individual competition, and the growth of health care enterprises. Measures of performance were now used to assess institutional effort, although the largely statistical techniques relied on measures less useful than convenient, such as number of beds or occupancy rates, and the direct application of performance measures to daily management was not common. The power and authority of the physician were still paramount and the doctor determined what should be done and to whom in the name of "quality" care. Ambulatory care, now recognized by the third-party payers, came into its own. Still, there were few priorities: planning was aimed at constraining proliferative growth, and organizations still largely reacted to their environments.

Network Medicine—The Third Era

The change in the health care environment that occurred over the last decade or so, coming gradually as it did, is marked by a general increase in the complexity and intractability of problems in the health industry. This new era, that of "network medicine" (Figure 1-3), is so called be-

Figure 1-3

Post-1975: Turbulent Environment
Costs + +
Change + +
Regulation +
Technology + +
Consumer demands +
Resources +

Era—Network Medicine
Many types of institutions
Many roles
Emphasis on extramural objectives—achieved results (health improvement)
Proactive
Variety of education
Education—continuous/value oriented
Service sectors—interdependent
Priorities set
Planning—long range, positive
Skills—diplomatic/collaboration/conflict resolution
Integration—intrinsic via collaboration, merger, regionalization, and coordination
Emphasis—total comprehensive care
Quality of life/quality of care determined by multiple publics

cause the increase in uncertainty and turbulence in the environment has been marked by the emergence of interdependent institutions for the first time, and, therefore, by a fundamental shift in values, structures, and dynamics.

The primary reason for this shift is that the environment is now scarce in resources and changing so dramatically and rapidly that information about it is remarkably uncertain. Federal deregulation promotes competition, while the states cap revenues. Consumers ask for more and ask more critically. The era is characterized by many alternative forms of service and/or service organizations with an expansion of the ambulatory sector, which is still not integrated fully. Integration, previously through informal referral and consultative networks, has become more intrinsic to institutions and is not left, as in other eras, essentially to chance. Integration is characterized by the emergence of wide varieties of multi-institutional systems and other forms of collaboration, such as mergers, consortia, regional networks, alliances, and super groups—a trend that will continue. For the first time, a cottage industry is maturing, is going through what industry did in the '20s, with massing of resources in major corporations. The for-profits led the way, the voluntaries are now, for the first time, matching them.

The increasing uncertainty of this era has resulted in more effective long-range planning, as well as the development of priorities by managers. Moreover, planning is now based on strategic considerations and tied directly to operations for ultimate effectiveness. In the era of network medicine, managers tap into different sets of skills and are no longer totally preoccupied with the interests of their own individual institutions, but are involved in larger institutional networks.

In past eras, health care institutions—hospitals in particular—were essentially buffered from the marketplace by the methods of reimbursement, in particular, cost reimbursement. Since hospitals got paid for what they did anyway, it did not matter what they did so long as the physician was kept reasonably happy. So the fact that most health care institutions did not have explicit strategies did not matter much. Competition among health care institutions has increased rapidly in this new era, however, as resources have become constrained and at the same time aggregated. While individual provider institutions used to compete (and then covertly) only with other providers in an immediate geographic vicinity—a neighborhood, city, or town—a group of institutions may now compete successfully not only within a state but an entire region. And in any large city today, there is increased local competition as new types of organizations arise. In the greater Boston area, 14 HMOs are competing essentially for the same population. The Visiting Nurse Association (VNA) of Denver, once the dominant if not sole provider of home health care, now competes with 22 home health agencies.

Essentially then, the health system appears to be moving in two general directions. The first is toward development of networks, usually geographically based, which integrate a wide variety of services and attempt to retain patients within them through cross-referral, or which attempt to retain patients on a captive basis through attractive financial mechanisms such as prepayment or the Preferred Provider Option (PPO). The second emerging system is usually not geographic and provides services to a wide variety of unrelated institutions (Figure 1-4). Both of these networks differ from traditional health care "systems" in which patients

Figure 1 - 4

Basic Types of Networks

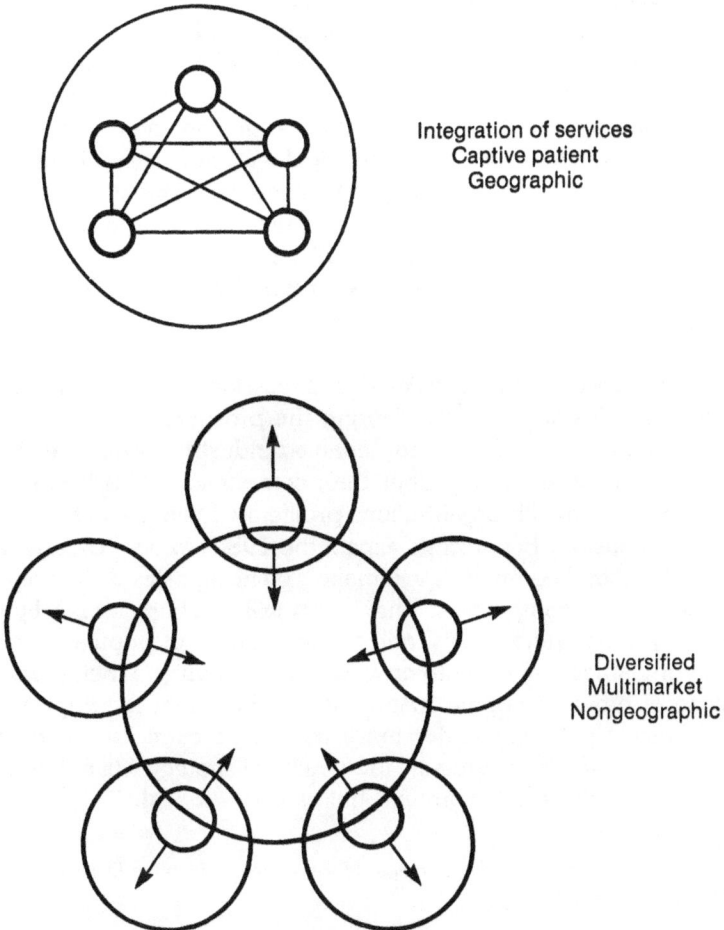

Integration of services
Captive patient
Geographic

Diversified
Multimarket
Nongeographic

moved among providers through informal or even "haphazard" referrals from one solo practitioner to another. Perhaps most importantly, provider institutions are adopting nontraditional views of the physician as a major source of patients and therefore the "marketing" agent. Institutions are now adopting industrial approaches to marketing, product definition, and the very concept of competition and competitive strategy.

In this third era—the era of uncertainty, of competition—the individual health care delivery organization must assess its competitive position amid a maze of events, a plethora of developments, an inundation of information. Competitive position is a function of the competitive forces with which the organization must contend. These, in turn, will be affected by the key general trends in the environment (see Chapter 3—scanning) which may influence the competitive forces differently for different organizations—and therefore the opportunities or threats posed by these trends must be considered in each unique instance.

While rational analysis is critical, it is the attitude and values of the key managers which will ultimately determine whether these managers see a particular constellation of trends and competitive forces as constituting a threat or an opportunity. To the extent that management is locked into a particular—traditional and somewhat rigid—way of seeing things and doing things, any change will be experienced as a threat rather than an opportunity. To the extent that management is open and willing to consider alternative possibilities, change will be experienced as providing opportunity. This issue, the enormous importance of world view in determining competitive outlook, will be discussed further in the last section of this chapter.

The conclusion derived from this discussion of the environment is echoed by industrial analysts.[1] During the prosperous 1950s and '60s, the rapid growth of the economy enabled industrial companies to focus their attention on demand rather than competition. This was the same period in which health organizations proliferated, since capital was available for expansion. Economists expect the 1980s to be a decade of slow growth. Industrial companies will make significant sales gains only at the expense of their competitors. The 1980s will be characterized by scarce resources, rising energy costs, and the leveling off of population growth. Thus, companies that hope to grow will have to pursue their gains at the expense of other companies. Analysts conclude that the importance of good strategic planning under these conditions cannot be overemphasized. As the decade progresses, the quality of strategy will determine not only a firm's prospects for growth, but its very survival.

---

[1] P. Stonich, ed., *Implementing Strategy: Making Strategy Happen* (New York: Ballinger Publishing, 1982).

Uncertainty and the Relevant Environment—
The Concept of Positioning

In Lawrence and Dyer's formulation, the environment can be characterized in two dimensions: the uncertainty of resource availability and the
uncertainty of information.[2] Figure 1-5 graphically shows that institutions
in the health field for the most part have moved from a relatively certain
environment to a highly uncertain one. Exceptions are those institutions
in rural areas or small towns, with little or no competition.

Competitive strategies are inevitable with resource scarcity and increased environmental complexity. Organizations must strategically ma-
neuver themselves in the industry to be favorably positioned for the future. Competitive strategy seeks to create options within limits, to identify

Figure 1-5

Evolution of the Environment

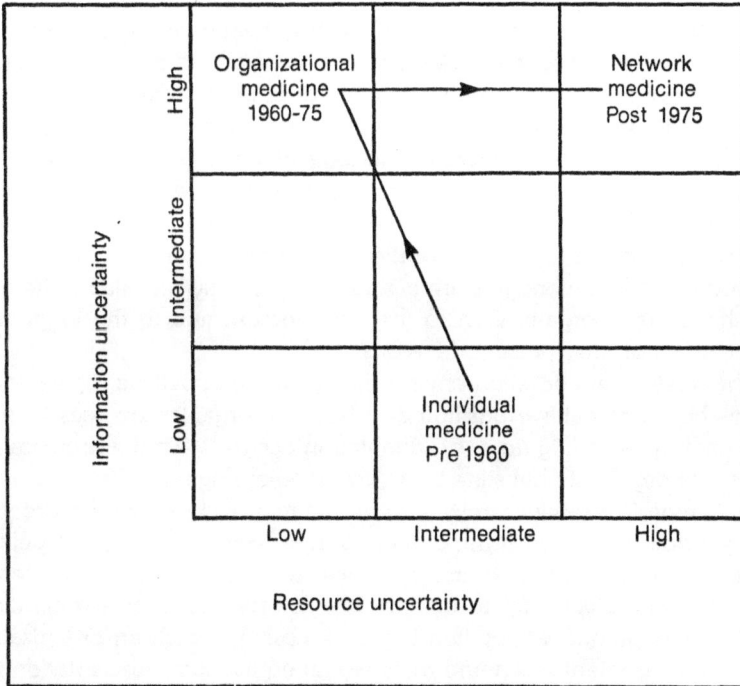

Source: Adapted from P. Lawrence and D. Dyer, *Renewing American Industry* (New York:
Free Press, 1983).

---

[2]P. Lawrence and D. Dyer, *Renewing American Industry* (New York: Free Press, 1983).

opportunities for growth and expansion within constraint, and to relate the organization to its environment. Positive and negative forces in the environment affect all organizations which operate in that environment; the essence of competitive strategy is to develop abilities appropriate to the particular organization, that enable it to deal with and advance in the environment.

The manager who thinks competitively must define and redefine what may be termed the "relevant environment(s)" for his or her organization. Typically, and certainly historically, managers of health care organizations narrowly delimited their relevant environments (the forces affecting them as well as their markets) and related services. Moreover, they tended to focus on equally narrow sets of behavior which were felt to determine successful operation in the relevant environment(s). In the short run, this enabled organizations to stabilize, and allowed managers some sense of controlled cause and effect in the interaction between organization and environment. The long-run effect, however, has too often been myopia—managers have treated the relevant environment as though it were the total environment, ignoring factors outside their "created" world. In this new era of network medicine, health care managers must redefine and reassess their relevant environments, in part by redefining what their organizations do now and could do in the future. Often, managers find themselves victims of the very procedures which they use to do and think about things, as well as the tools they use to measure what the organization does. These processes can get in the way of adapting to future needs when they become so entrenched as to be inflexible. A reasonable adaptation to the environment in the short-run can hinder future adaptation unless managers are careful to constantly reevaluate the relationship of their organization to the environment and to the longer-run implications of their present decisions.

The relationship between environmental and competitive forces, then, affects both competitive position and how the organization sees its relevant environment (Figure 1-6); adaptation occurs when the organization adjusts its organizational state to a desired level (Figure 1-7).

A change in perceived relevant environment will usually then require corresponding changes in the organization as well as in all its competitive strategy, for the organization's competitive position will have altered. Lawrence and Dyer refer to this process as organizational *readaptation*. While organizational adaptation is the process by which an organization and its environment reach and maintain an equilibrium, readaptation is a form of that adaptation in which the organization and its relevant environment interact and evolve toward new exchanges that are more acceptable to the internal and external stakeholders. The process is evidenced by continuing high levels of innovation, efficiency, and member involvement. Readaptation is distinct from adaptation in much the same way

Figure 1-6

Forces Affecting Competitive Position

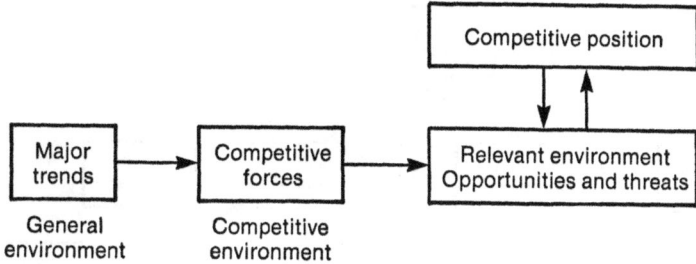

```
                                    ┌──────────────────────┐
                                    │ Competitive position │
                                    └──────────────────────┘
                                         ↓        ↑
┌──────────┐      ┌──────────────┐   ┌──────────────────────────┐
│  Major   │ ───► │ Competitive  │──►│  Relevant environment    │
│  trends  │      │   forces     │   │ Opportunities and threats│
└──────────┘      └──────────────┘   └──────────────────────────┘
  General           Competitive
environment         environment
```

Figure 1-7

Adaptation

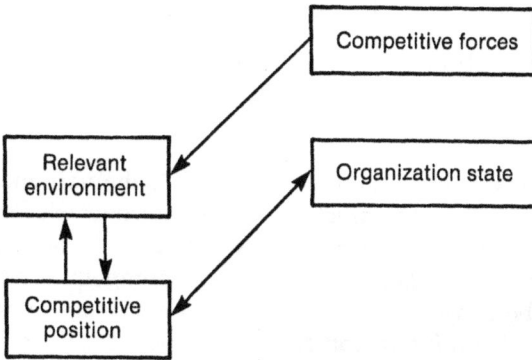

```
                              ┌──────────────────┐
                              │ Competitive forces│
                              └──────────────────┘
                                     ╲
        ┌──────────────┐          ┌──────────────────┐
        │  Relevant    │◄─        │ Organization state│
        │ environment  │          └──────────────────┘
        └──────────────┘             ╱
           ↑    ↓                   ╱
        ┌──────────────┐◄──────────
        │ Competitive  │
        │  position    │
        └──────────────┘
```

that research is distinct from search; the former is a continuous and systematic process.

Organizational strategy refers to an organization's definition of its goals, and the relevant environment delineates an area or market in which to pursue these goals. Strategic decisions will determine the internal arrangements best suited to meeting desired ends (goals) in the relevant environment (Figure 1-8). Organizations which have adapted to a historical context, a past relevant environment facing a changing relevant environment, must readapt not just to the present but to their projection of some *future* context if readaptation is to be successful and enduring. Otherwise, they will continually have to change with each minor environmental shift. Actions taken in the present are then departures from the past, oriented to some (perhaps) ill-defined future, and only having

Figure 1 - 8

Readaptation

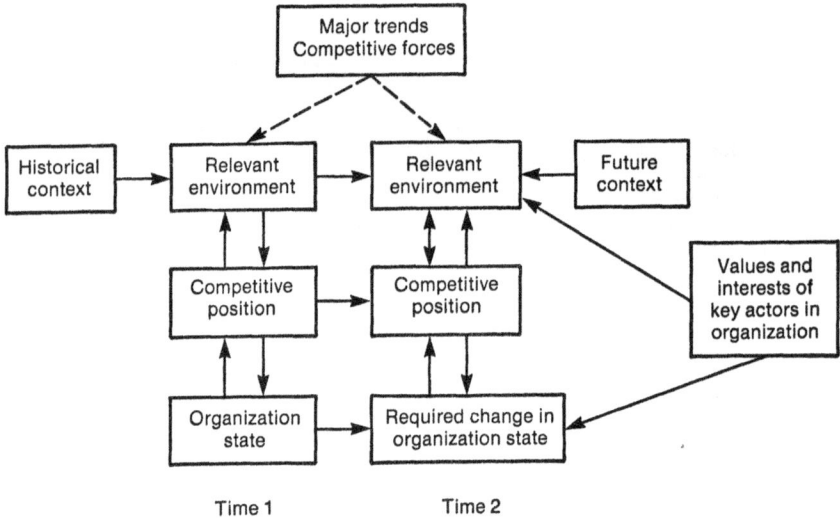

meaning in these contextual relationships. It is the very momentum and comfort of the past and imprecision of the future which fosters so much discomfort and reluctance to change. An organization readapts by engaging in positioning activities to regain its lost competitive advantage. But these cannot be considered out of context, or they are without meaning.

The historical and future contexts determine attitude and resistance as well as justification. Look at, for example, consolidation. Is it necessary to achieve goals, and might it be acceptable, given, for instance, a historical context which included a strong desire for ownership? One might consolidate activities to help people learn to work together, i.e., to get their values to change, to save money, or to position the organization for a new venture. But there is always a trade-off in any positioning activity. For example, with consolidation, one may get economies of scale, but at the cost of moving the activity further from the market.

Positioning activities, then, are the link between past and future (Figure 1-9). With much uncertainty about both resources and information, knowledge of where to find what becomes central. This is *scanning* (Chapter 3). A way of reducing information uncertainty is to know more about less—a result of successful *product market analysis* (Chapter 4). Resources can be aggregated when scarce through *collaboration* (Chapter 5), which also provides the support for more sophisticated scanning.

Figure 1-9

The Role of Positioning

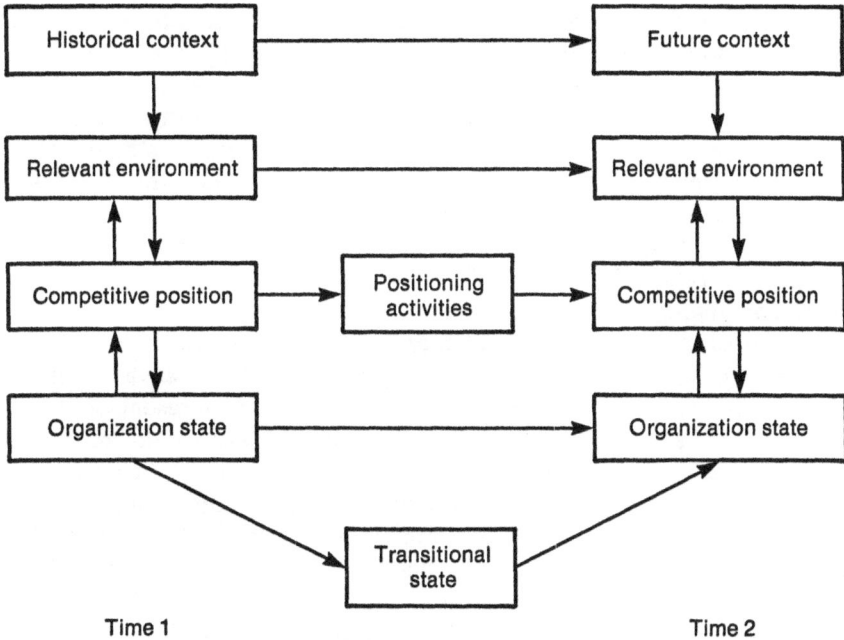

Organizing resources more efficiently to address product/market segments through *restructuring* (Chapter 6) also conserves a scarce commodity. Finally, internal conflicts about direction and purpose consume resources, necessitating the *management of physicians* (Chapter 7) if organizational redirection is to occur. These positioning activities are required to bring about readaptation.

Readaptation is a special form of adaptation marked by the repeated discovery of ways to introduce innovations, while maintaining or enhancing efficiencies and member involvement. Enacting an effective competitive strategy is a form of readaptation. Efficiency refers to the ratio of inputs to outputs. All organizations will operate most effectively where maximum output is derived from each input used. In health care, efficiency may be gained by addressing services (products) more precisely to markets, or by restructuring resources through corporate reorganization.

Innovations are new ways of seeing. An innovation is a new idea which a set of people with a stake in the organization have found appropriate to the organization's goals and have adopted for regular use. By definition, an innovation disturbs the established order. In the short run, by promoting unestablished ways of doing things, innovations can be in conflict with efficiency; however, in the long run, innovations can be very complementary and are necessary for readaptation. Sell what we do well to others—the shared service concept—is an innovation.

Finally, member involvement describes the extent to which all levels and categories of an organization's employees identify themselves with the organization and share a fate in it. In other words, the extent to which organizational changes do or do not alienate persons with a vested interest in the organization. How, for example, can physicians be encouraged to be more productive and less cost inducing when their interests may be in conflict with a hospital's? The set of positioning activities and the process of creating competitive strategic action are intended to address these readaptive issues. The three indicators—efficiency, innovation, and member involvement—are taken by Lawrence and Dyer as measures of the success with which an organization is able to readapt to its current environment or adapt to newly defined relevant environments.

The Visiting Nurse Association (VNA) of Denver represents a good example of the choices involved in defining a new relevant environment and in developing new alternative strategies that will result in readaptation. Having in the past provided a wide range of home care services through its monopoly market, the organization suddenly faces extensive competition on all fronts from 22 agencies. Can it continue to be all things to all people, or should it focus upon a specific market segment? The definition of its business in the past has been heavily oriented to home nursing care. But the nature of the needs of its market suggests that a broader range of services is required than those which can be provided solely by nurses: occupational therapies, rehabilitation therapies, physical therapies, etc. Moreover, the efficient use of these other skills suggests that their provision in the home is not optimal. Ambulatory patients requiring a wide range of therapies might be more efficiently treated in day-care centers judiciously placed throughout the Denver area. Should the business be redefined as one which provides to communities a broad range of nonmedical care both at home and through day-care centers? Should the VNA focus upon the relatively easy cases requiring little expertise for a brief time, or upon the complex cases requiring much care over time? Resolving these decisions may make the difference between success and failure for the VNA.

In many ways, an organization is analogous to a human personality. It contains sets of attributes or capacities as well as shortcomings. While it may be comfortable in its old habits, it can learn new ways, rediscover old forgotten abilities. Shifts in the relevant environment may call upon one or the other—but old habits die hard, and this is the subject of the next section.

Uncertainty, Values, and the Need for Change

Foster: *Do you know what I saw once in the desert, in the*
Australian desert? A man walking along carrying two
umbrellas. Two umbrellas. In the outback.

Spooner: *Was it raining?*

Foster: *No it was a beautiful day. I nearly asked him what he was*
up to but I changed my mind.

Spooner: *Why?*

Foster: *Well, I decided he must be some kind of lunatic. I*
thought he would only confuse me.

Harold Pinter

The types of changes described thus far seem profound and multidimensional, and they are. They involve seeing and doing things differently. Historically, health institutions have been accidental aggregations of activities which have become so bundled together that the institution has become sacrosanctly synonymous with the activity set, e.g., a hospital. Health institutions, be they teaching, service, or research oriented, have been also fiercely independent entities, whether this was necessary or not. An essential argument made in this book is that there are economic and social forces changing the environment in which individuals live and organizations function. The environment, as it becomes increasingly complex and unpredictable, places demands on individuals and organizations. To function effectively, not only must new strategies be developed which guide organizational behavior, but corresponding shifts in values, in attitudes, in total world view must occur. In other words, a paradigm shift is called for. Kuhn argues that occasionally there comes along a kind of science that changes the rules, which he calls "paradigmatic science."[3] A paradigm is, in a way, a world as well as a world view. Paradigms guide behavior by providing a model as well as a set of rules about the "accepted" way in which things are done.

Health care institutions, like all organizations, work according to paradigms.[4] Health professionals practicing their technologies are organized by their tasks and structured into paradigmatic relationships which are kept dynamic by the way they are measured and controlled. Managers of health care organizations develop organizational policies and strategies based, in part, on personal values and beliefs which generally spring from

---

[3]T. Kuhn, *The Structure of Scientific Revolutions*, vol. 11 (Chicago: University of Chicago Press, 1970).

[4]A. Sheldon, *Managing Change and Collaboration in the Health Field* (Cambridge, Mass.: Oelgeschlager, Gunn and Hain, 1979).

broader societal expectations as well as from traditional paradigms about cause and effect in the industry. Physician-patient relationships have a paradigmatic basis, as do the relationships between physicians and other nonmedical staff. Similarly, there are attitudes and beliefs strongly grounded in paradigm which have historically driven health care institutions to seek autonomy whenever possible, defined the types of services which should be offered in alternative provider setting, and in other ways giving a distinct character to the health industry. All of this is directed toward some end called "order" or "status quo" which is sometimes explicit, sometimes implicit. The point, however, is that the institutions and professionals in the health sector share certain values and attitudes which correspond to prevailing paradigms.

A paradigm, a world view, has a not surprising stubbornness, not surprising when you consider how many people's careers and lives are rooted in it. It is not surprising, then, that relevant environments, being ways in which organizations perceive the environments around them, have an intransigence that is beyond rationality. As people don't want to see changes that will distress them, so organizations are blinkered to unwelcome information. If you don't ask questions, you won't get confused.

The need for a paradigmatic change or shift comes about under two circumstances. If an organization becomes closed and stops adapting, at some point it will get out of touch with its environment. When this becomes significant enough, a paradigmatic shift is necessary. Second, and more commonly, paradigmatic shifts occur when the environment to which an organization has been responding adaptively, but simply, reaches a point that requires multidimensional readaptation on the part of the organization. In other words, paradigmatic change involves a change in several dimensions at once. But most fundamentally, it requires a change in the way the organization's world functions and sees the universe outside it.

As world views, paradigms are rooted in values and beliefs which determine how issues are perceived and what people do; thus it is arguable that the persistence of values which were appropriate to the previous eras of medicine are bedeviling attempts to solve problems in this new era. For example, the physician has always been dominant, sacrosanct, and self-governing in the health sector. At one time, this may have been both appropriate and desirable; however, the autonomy of the physician is no longer totally appropriate. The physician determines costs through treatment decisions. In an era of constrained resources, the physician who continues to make treatment decisions in the absence of efficiency concerns (appropriate in previous eras when values supported heroic medical efforts with no thought for resource use) is destroying his or her organization. Similarly, while teamwork and collaboration were a matter of discretion in the era of organizational medicine, they have become a matter of necessity in the era of network medicine. Yet these behaviors are all the more difficult because they not only represent a departure from past values, but are encouraged by outmoded incentive mechanisms. The development of new value sets which support strategies for conflict resolution becomes critical to the development of new competitive strategies.

In short, the depth and pervasiveness of changes in the new environment may demand paradigm change consistent with the need for new strategies to control a rapidly changing health system. In the new environment, for example, control is furthered by collaboration and integration. The key to these behaviors lies in an attitude and value shift from that of a single institution orientation to that of a network-oriented set of shared values. Values must also be concerned not with medical heroics but with the provision of care that is responsibly directed to the quality of patients' lives and to the use of society's scarce resources. Individual organizations cannot be expected to readapt successfully to a rapidly changing environment simply through their own direct action. Successful readaptation must be accompanied by the emergence of new values that have significance for all members of the field, as a way of coping with the uncertainty and complexity of change.

The two keys to paradigm change are the efficacy of the new paradigm (and sterility of the old) and the change in values and beliefs of the organization's members. There are three types of paradigmatic shift which have particular relevance for the collaborative process: (1) side by side, (2) transformation, and (3) supraparadigm.

1. Side by side   The new paradigm emerges alongside the old, which continues to exist. The prerequisite for successful change is the buffering—physically, organizationally, and fiscally—of each from the other.

2. Transformation   Transformation is lengthy, and value and belief change are crucial predecessors of any later structural changes, as is repudiation of the old paradigm. The new cannot be entertained until the old is moribund, if not defunct. This requires:

a.   Condemnation through a careful process of confronting consequences. The old may need an extra push (by neglecting, for instance, to institute normal change) before a shift is entertained.
b.   Attitude change through presentation of data and, if necessary, changing people in critical roles.
c.   A transitional organization in which steps a and b may be accomplished and which, since it will replace the old before the new is there to be experienced, must be a trusted process and structure.
d.   A mourning process for what is gone.

3. Supraparadigm   In purest form, the supraparadigm contains, but transcends, the old paradigms. In other words, managers must offer a positive vision (rather than, as in side by side and transformation, something to replace something else that does not work).

Finally, it is probably true that all three types of change are distinctly helped by the existence of a leader who transcends the warring or failing paradigms and is not identified with one side or another except, as in the last case, with something above all.

Summary

The environment has, in the last quarter century, been characterized by an increasingly rapid rate of change in many dimensions. It has become extraordinarily complex and uncertain, especially in the areas of information and resource availability. The era of *individual medicine,* prior to 1960, was one of a simple, slowly changing environment characterized by the individual practitioner practicing largely in isolation. The next 15 years or so was the era of *organizational medicine,* as the modal size of health care institutions grew rapidly in a relatively resource rich environment. The last 10 years have been turbulent, with resources more constrained and competition emphasized. In such an era, it is argued that institutions must compete for information and resources and can only do so successfully if they work together as well as compete. This is termed the era of *network medicine.* Organizations which were adapted to prior eras must now readapt to this new environment. They do so through engaging in positioning activities which enable them to gain competitive advantage. This new era not only requires strategies, but successful competitive strategies, entailing an alteration in basic values. The acquisition of new shared values and the juggling of competition and collaboration simultaneously require new world views, new skills, and new kinds of managers.

The Model of Competitive Strategy

A fool must now and then be right, by chance.
William Cowper

In this chapter, the model sketched in Chapter 1 is filled out. The concepts of general and competitive strategy are discussed, and the process described. The general environmental trends and competitive forces that create a relevant environment are detailed. Evaluation of adaptation is then the issue. This involves understanding and assessing competitive position and performance, and reconsidering strategy, goals, and objectives as they determine tasks and, thus, organizational state. The measures of competitive position and performance and the characteristics of organizational state are reviewed. The basic questions are: How well are you adapted to the relevant environment? If poorly, what must you change? If it has changed, what must you do to readapt? Are you defining your business(es) correctly, or should it (they) be redefined? The two last parts of the chapter then deal with positioning activities and competitive strategies in brief—these are discussed further in the later chapters of the book.

What Is Strategy Development?

Strategy development is the process by which managers make two major decisions: the overall goals/direction toward which their organizations will be moving in the future, and the way(s) in which the organization will pursue activities towards those ends. Essentially, a strategy is a broad formula which systematically delineates organizational goals, policies needed to achieve goals, and definitions of how the organization will operate pursuant to its goals and policies. Managers may use different terms for these concepts. *Ends* are synonymous with the goals to which an organization strives, and *means* are the policies by which it seeks to get there; other terms often used are *mission statement,* for goal, and *tactics,* for means or policies. The essential notion of strategy, however, is contained in the clear *delineation of ends versus means to obtain ends.*

A strategy must be founded on organizational goal statements, which are very broad definitions of purpose, the more specific level of desired objectives (which may be expressed in economic as well as noneconomic terms), and the projected ability to operate in the environment. Goal statements may address, for example, desired levels of profitability, future leadership in the field, community responsiveness, innovation in medical practice, growth, increased market share, etc. Goals may be stated explicitly by management, or the organization may have only implicit goals which are part of a "general future direction." Goals involve judgments about fluctuating and uncertain factors and may reflect desire as much as rationality, values as much as logic.

Effective managers typically announce only a few broad goals from the top while encouraging staff in their institutions to propose other goals and while allowing still others to emerge from informal processes. Goals express pinnacles for an organization or, if you will, the dreams and aspirations of the organization's managers and governing boards. Unfortunately, goals per se are often too vague to have day-to-day meaning or to offer operational directives; therefore, goal statements should generally be translated by managers into objectives and/or milestones—quantifiable targets which have clearly attached behaviors that must be undertaken to reach the target. For example, a hospital's goal may be to become the "major oncology center in its region." This is a tall order. Moreover, in and of itself, the goal gives no indication of how it might be achieved or even what is meant by "major." Objectives and milestones translate this goal into measurable and manageable tasks: increase our hospital's annual rate of admissions to the oncology service 20 percent by the end of the next fiscal year; recruit three nationally renowned oncologists to our hospital by fiscal year 1986; increase the number of residency training slots in this specialty by four over the next fiscal year; purchase X pieces of equipment by fiscal year 1988, etc. Based on these objectives, the hospital administrator and senior staff can develop a specific set of interim activities that will be needed to meet each objective and incrementally move the hospital towards its goal. Some organization's managers—for example, the administrator of a small community hospital located in an isolated geographic area—can afford to be less specific in articulating both goals and objectives and still develop an effective strategy. However, most organizations—for example, large (teaching) hospitals in major urban centers, competing with numerous hospitals and other health care institutions—need clear, objective statements for effective strategy. Regardless of the specificity of goal statements, the concept of strategy refers first and foremost to a plan which guides the overall behavior and operation of the organization towards specified end results.

Closely related to the goal-oriented dimension of organizational strategy is its second dimension: strategy represents a conscious decision by management to *review past behaviors, policies, and operations and, if required, to evolve towards new ones.*

Interestingly, this must be the case even if management's goals are to maintain an organizational status quo. Because an organization's operating environment rarely remains constant, it may be incumbent upon management to follow the advice of di Lampedusa that one must change to remain the same.[1] Even during the eras of individual and organizational medicine when the rate of change was relatively slow, the environment did not remain totally static. In the highly turbulent and competitive environment of the current era, network medicine, managers must realize that even no-growth goals require some growth if the status quo is to be maintained. Hospitals, health centers, and other providers face increasingly constrained (capped) revenues while costs increase. With no strategy to increase revenues or reduce costs, both of which will require that the organization make some changes, the net result is more likely to be organizational regression than maintenance of the status quo.

The strategic process can thus be viewed as anticipatory management and, indeed, initiation of organizational change to prepare for the future. Strategy is intended to deal not with the present, or it would be outmoded before it was realized, but with a probable future that, ironically, might never be. In developing strategies for their institutions, managers must look objectively at the institution's present competitive position: how it has been operating in the past, where it should be headed in the future, and how it is going to get there. Managers must then assess the consequences and incremental effects of their present decisions vis-à-vis movement towards future goals, as well as the resistance these decisions may generate as they move away from a cherished past. It is important to

---

[1] G. di Lampedusa, *The Leopard* (New York: Penguin Books, 1955).

recognize that each and every decision should not and *cannot* move the organization towards its goals in quantum leaps and bounds. Rather, present choices made by managers can best be given meaning and perspective by representing changes from past behavior and promoting future, goal-directed movement of the organization. Strategy deals not so much with present management decisions as with the futurity of present decisions.[2] Strategy also involves judgment about best courses and likely consequences. Only the actions taken to fulfill specific objectives have an irrefutable logic, and even that can be overtaken by events.

To answer the question, "Where is this institution going or where should it go?" requires that managers answer other questions: (1) What are the major external factors that do and will influence the institution? (2) What opportunities and/or problems are these factors likely to present? (3) How can the institution best capitalize on any anticipated opportunities while at the same time minimizing the impact of anticipated problems? The challenge of good strategy development is to answer these questions and answer them well. In today's environment, all health care organizations should develop coordinated answers to these questions.

Historically, most health care institutions have engaged in planning processes which occurred implicitly, through the activities of various departments or units. Left to their own activities, however, these departments have generally pursued strategies dictated by their own orientations and professional interests. The "sum" of these "parts" has not always resulted in sound corporate strategy. For example, the New York City Health and Hospitals Corporation's senior staff could be pursuing potentially conflicting goals. The president has publicized the deemphasis of tertiary care and promoted the concept of becoming the family doctor for New York's poor. Other senior staff recognize that, to maximize revenues, their hospitals should increase the richness of their case mix and do more complex procedures. Carried to their extremes, these approaches could result in quite different, possibly incompatible strategies. Positioning activities, as discussed below, must be harmonized, even if ultimate goals remain somewhat obscure.

Chapter 1 stated that the uncertainty and turbulence of the health care environment demand the development of an explicit and *competitive* organizational strategy. Changes in regulatory and reimbursement policies, resource availability, and complexity of information necessitate a self-consciously planned approach to change if managers are going to manage their institutions effectively. In addition, reduced resource availability and other newly imposed constraints facing health care organizations require that managers also address issues of competition in the industry: What is

---

[2]P. F. Drucker, *Management Tasks, Responsibilities, Practices* (New York: Harper & Row, 1973).

driving the newly heightened competitive force among providers of care? How will the industry evolve? Who are my organization's chief competitors and what are they likely to do in the future? How can we be best positioned in the industry to compete successfully in the long run?

The Strategic Process

Traditional approaches to strategy development imply a separation between strategy formulation and enactment. You think, then do. In fact, this is not what happens or should happen. Organizations generally do, then articulate. Quinn is the foremost proponent of this incremental process.[3] The process, it must be emphasized, is not an end in itself, hence the emphasis in this book on action.

Formulating an effective competitive strategy requires more than innovative thinking, good data, and expert analysis of the environment. Whether and how well a strategic alternative can be executed by the organization must be the operating context for strategy formulation. Managers must recognize that their organization's needs will not be met by strategies based only on external factors (environmental context). Many barriers to making a strategy happen are, in fact, found within the organization itself. Failing to consider the "inhouse" issues related to implementation of strategy will doom in advance strategies that, in other respects, are well conceived. Hence, the emphasis here is on understanding the historical context, i.e., the world that the organization has created and may be attached to.

Whatever the approach, the same issues are considered important by most authors, though perhaps labeled differently and in different order.[4-7]

All approaches propose looking at:

- What the organization is now doing.
- The industry
- The competitors ———— as they present opportunities and threats.
- Society
- The organization's strengths and weaknesses.

---

[3]J. B. Quinn, *Strategies for Change: Logical Incrementalism* (Homewood, Ill.: Richard D. Irwin, 1980).

[4]M. Porter, *Competitive Strategy: Techniques for Analyzing Industries and Competitors* (New York: Free Press, 1980).

[5]Quinn, *Strategies for Change.*

[6]*Business Policy as a Field of Study*, Harvard University School of Business, ICCH No. 378-291 (Cambridge, Mass., 1978).

[7]Drucker, *Management Tasks.*

and then considering whether the existing strategy, as implemented, can continue to work, and if not, what the alternatives are and which should be chosen.

Quinn's statement of the incremental approach suggests that competitive strategy is rarely derived from a totally formal planning process or a management-by-objectives approach, but rather, from an iterative, largely political process wherein consensus building is critical, and precise beginnings and endings are hard to delineate. Far from being haphazard, this can be an effective management technique for improving and integrating the analytic and behavioral aspects of strategy formulation. In summary, then, the organization must:

Establish a systematic basis for relating the allocation of scarce resources to the realities of changing markets.

Promote continual adaptation of the institutional mission and program structure to changing regulatory, market, and other environmental conditions.

Attempt to preserve financial viability in the face of scarce resources.

Enhance management's control of change through tactical decision making.

Increase understanding of the operating environment and, therefore, of staff competence at proactive decision making.

Competitive strategy must be purposeful (goal directed), politically astute, and defined in terms of a relevant environment. Because strategy is generally formulated over a long period, the process is rarely completely orderly, rationally predictable, or totally internally consistent. Managers must respond flexibly and opportunistically to new threats, crises, or opportunities which could not have been foreseen at the time the competitive strategy was initiated. Developing such strategy is both science and craft, requiring a subtle balance of vision, entrepreneurship, and political acumen.

Quinn characterizes the process in terms of a series of strategic subsystems from which emerges a holistic organizational strategy. While, at first, the processes used appear to be disjointed or "muddling," they, in fact, are strongly logical and consistent. Effective strategies emerge from a series of strategic formulation subsystems, each involving somewhat different sets of players, information needs, and time imperatives. Each subsystem attacks a particular issue in a disciplined way, yet each is incremental and somewhat opportunistic in its formulation. While the logic underlying each subsystem's strategy is powerful, the timing of each is different. Because of this, the total enterprise's strategy has to address the interactions of all the subsystems' strategies and, of necessity, is derived from an approach he describes as "logical incrementalism."

The steps are: (1) establishing systematic means to help sense new strategic needs well in advance; (2) building awareness and legitimizing viewpoints about perceived new options; (3) broadening support and building psychological comfort levels for action; (4) starting and stimulating ad hoc programs to generate partial solutions; (5) avoiding early identification with specific solutions to maintain flexibility, organizational decentralization, and personal motivation of lower echelons; (6) managing political coalitions to develop and crystallize consensus as it emerges; (7) getting individuals to identify personally with intended strategies; and (8) actively shaping accepted proposals in patterns which support goals that may be only broadly conceived at first, but evolve interactively along with action alternatives, toward more precise ultimate commitments.

Crises can collapse time frames or cause abrupt shifts in an organization's direction, but most strategic decisions in large enterprises emerge as a process of continuous, evolving, political consensus building, with no precise beginning or end. Quinn concludes that managing the generation and evolution of this consensus is one of the true arts of management, calling for the best practices both of the behavioral sciences and of theories of decision making.

It is time to return to the model sketched in Chapter 1. The organization must review and consider the historical context as regards:

Environmental trends.
Competitive forces.
The relevant environment it defined.
Its competitive position and performance historically and now.
Its goals, objectives, and strategy, and the tasks deriving from these.
Its organizational state, as fitting the tasks.

It should assess how well its past adaptation succeeded and will endure as the organization projects the future context:

Environmental trends.
Competitive forces.
Its future relevant environment.
Its future competitive position and likely future performance.

The organization should then consider whether it should and can readapt by:

Redefining the business it is in.
Redirecting its goals, objectives, strategy, and therefore tasks, and shifting its organizational state to fit those altered tasks.

through taking and making:

Positioning actions, separately but harmoniously.
Organizational change.

Even if the relevant environment and/or competitive position have not altered, adaptation may still not have occurred because of inadequacies in strategy or implementation. Change will still then be indicated. Relevant environment change may be missed or ignored because the organization wants to believe the past will endure. This is a good place to involve consultants who can confront key actors as inside staff cannot. Judicious redefinition of business(es) will alter the relevant environment (and the competitive forces) radically. Is the Harvard Community Health Plan in the insurance business, the HMO business, the preventive health business, the health delivery business, the consulting business, or all of them? Is it competing with Blue Cross and Aetna, with Bay State Independent Practice Association and Tufts HMO, or with the local hospitals? Is the VNA in ambulatory nursing, home health care, or community care?

Environmental Trends

These trends are important as they affect competitive forces, and therefore competitive performance.

It is important to consider major *demographic trends.* What shifts are occurring generally and in the market area? What out- and in-migrations are happening? Will this affect the proportion of self-paying patients, or will new migrants present particular disease patterns or social needs? Both St. James and St. Mary's hospitals in Newark, New Jersey, face shifts in their ethnic markets from second-generation Irish and Italian to Portugese and Haitian. These shifts involve linguistic, cultural, and financial issues (the Haitian immigrants are poorer). The very sick and very old represent a major new development and an as yet unsolved problem, especially for HMOs.

Technological trends are also critical. Increasingly, health institutions may only remain competitive if they can provide the same technological capacity as their competitors. Thus, even the smallest hospital now needs to have a CAT scanner. And a larger one "must" have an NMR. Because of the increasing expense of technology, the cost of competition is constantly being raised. Moreover, new technology may make possible the existence of new forms of health care and, so, new competition. The development of noninvasive diagnostic techniques, for example, now makes it possible for many diagnostic workups to be done in ambulatory care rather than an in-patient setting, allowing free-standing diagnostic clinics to spring up. Communications technology now makes it possible to deliver monitoring and safety services to the elderly at home through interactive cable systems.

Social and life style changes are also important. Consumer attitudes in the health system have changed rapidly and patients now demand more

Competitive Strategy Model

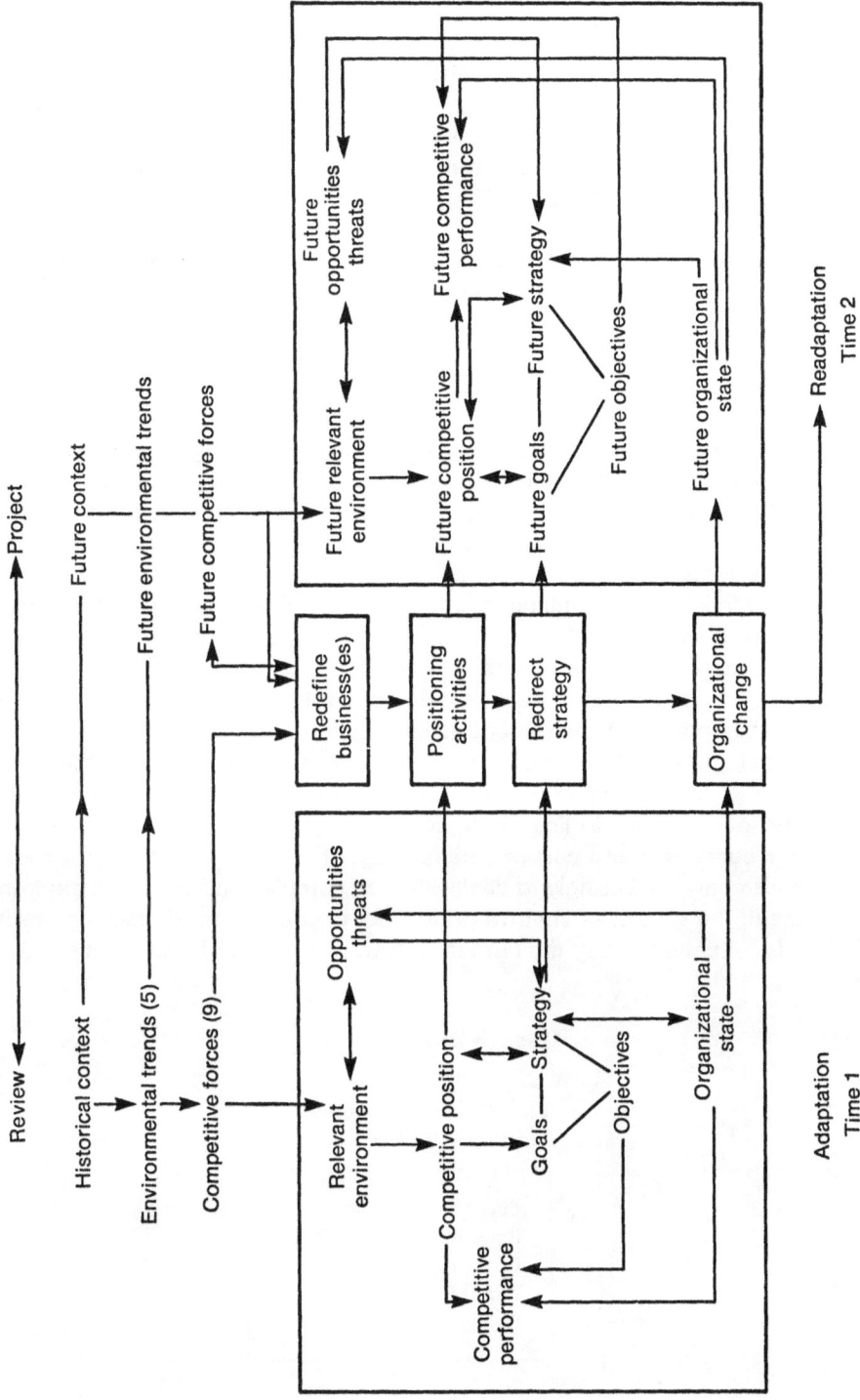

Review ← → Project

Historical context → Future context

Environmental trends (5) → Future environmental trends

Competitive forces (9) → Future competitive forces

Adaptation
Time 1

Readaptation
Time 2

Time 1 box:

Relevant environment

Opportunities threats

Competitive position

Competitive performance

Goals

Strategy

Objectives

Organizational state

Center boxes:

Redefine business(es)

Positioning activities

Redirect strategy

Organizational change

Time 2 box:

Future relevant environment

Future opportunities threats

Future competitive position

Future competitive performance

Future goals

Future strategy

Future objectives

Future organizational state

self-determination as well as more opportunities to control their own care. They are more critical and more articulate about the attributes of care they value. There is a greater concern and need for health-promoting activities, as people have become preoccupied with healthy lifestyles and alarmed about the environment. These trends present an opportunity for those institutions willing and able to offer programs responsive to the needs.

Economic trends should also be examined. For example, with economic recession comes unemployment; with computers and robotics, quite probably continuing high levels of unemployment. The unemployed have higher physical and mental illness rates, and are less able to pay for care if their benefits run out. This affects product market value in that such patients may represent a loss to the hospital. The rising costs of employee benefits are resulting in employers seeking ways to diminish their burden by controlling health care costs either directly or through new types of buyer relationship such as Preferred Provider Options (PPOs), or even by getting into the health field themselves. Simultaneously, however, governmental concerns with rising costs to Medicare and Medicaid are resulting in an attempt to shift the burden of these costs to the private sector.

A thorough environmental survey should also consider *regulatory* and *political trends*. These are obviously numerous, but three may be selected as examples from the current health environment. First, the government is deregulating, thus making more competition possible. At the same time, states are increasingly concerned with the costs of medical care and are seeking ways to limit these costs through efforts such as prospective reimbursement and cost or revenue caps. Finally, as health organizations collaborate increasingly to deal with their complex and uncertain environment, the specter of antitrust draws ever closer. Will most teaching hospitals continue to carry the burden of teaching costs and thus be at a disad-

Figure 2-2

**Five Major Environmental
Trends to Watch**

Social and lifestyle.
Regulatory/political/legal.
Economic.
Technological.
Demographic.

vantage in cost competition (e.g., for PPOs)? Will there be a physician glut? These are all issues that must be watched closely for their potential consequences. The environmental trends are summarized in Figure 2-2.

How to get information on and analyze the trends and forces will be addressed in Chapter 3 on scanning.

Decide: to succumb to the preponderance of one set of influences over another set.

Ambrose Bierce

The Competitive Forces

It is important to try to assess the likely moves that the existing competition may make. In the past, this has not been too difficult to do within the health system, since health institutions tended to be relatively slowly changing, predictable, and disinclined to make dramatic moves. However, as acquisitions and mergers become common and health organizations spin off management capabilities as separate businesses, competitive moves have become more rapid, more aggressive, and more common. Potential competitors to health care providers now may come from organizations not in the industry but easily able to overcome entry barriers. A number of industrial companies have recently entered aspects of the health field that they deem to be lucrative, such as home health or dialysis. These are often for-profit organizations previously either outside the health field completely or outside that particular market. Mergers or acquisitions, by increasing the resources available to an institution, often enable organizations to compete in far wider markets and suddenly to become competitive with former noncompetitors. In the South Clinic's case (Chapter 8), for example, competition for the regional patients had traditionally existed only among the hospitals in the clinic's own city. (The clinic did compete with institutions in distant cities for international tertiary care patients.) However, a recent merger in a city some 400 miles away resulted in the formation of a 2,000-bed giant which is now competing directly for many of South Clinic's regional patients.

Finally, among health organizations, competition is no longer simply for patients or for physicians (who are the essential marketers for patients), but for the variety of services—clinical or management—that health organizations both need and may provide. This type of competition is extraordinarily complex and will be discussed below in relation to the formulation of strategy.

What determines competition among organizations? Porter identifies five forces which determine the strength of competition in any industry and which are, therefore, crucial factors from the point of view of strategy formulation.[8] These forces are:

Entry.

Threat of substitution.

Rivalry among traditional competitors.

Bargaining power of suppliers.

Bargaining power of buyers.

Add to Porter's list four other forces which affect the strength of competition in the health industry:

Management services—strength and availability.

Clinical services—strength and availability.

Access to capital markets.

Effects of reimbursement systems.

A composite model of the competitive forces and their interactions can be seen in Figure 2–3. Below, each force is discussed individually. It is important to understand that all nine forces must be considered jointly to determine the intensity of industry competition. The strongest forces govern the nature and strength of competition, provide the relevant environment, create the competitive position, and are the most critical for strategy development. This modification/expansion of Porter's model reflects the fact that within different industries, different forces take prominence in fueling the nature and strength of organizational competition. The model is made more relevant to the health care industry through the addition of salient forces which are less generalizable to other industries but have strong implications for competition among providers of health care.

New *entrants* may come into a market from any of a number of directions and may enter the patient-care or non-patient-care segments of the market. In the patient-care segment, a hospital may decide to acquire or build a new ambulatory care center within another hospital's market area to "steal" referrals and support its primary care referral base. Hospital groups, especially those originating from for-profit companies, may acquire or build: a referral base, relationships with secondary or tertiary care institutions, and/or free-standing clinical services. An HMO, either autonomous or attached to an existing institution, may spring up. The biggest fear of existing hospitals in a market area is that the area will be invaded by the for-profits or by major new groupings of collaborating in-

---

[8]Porter, *Competitive Strategy.*

Figure 2-3

Competitive Forces

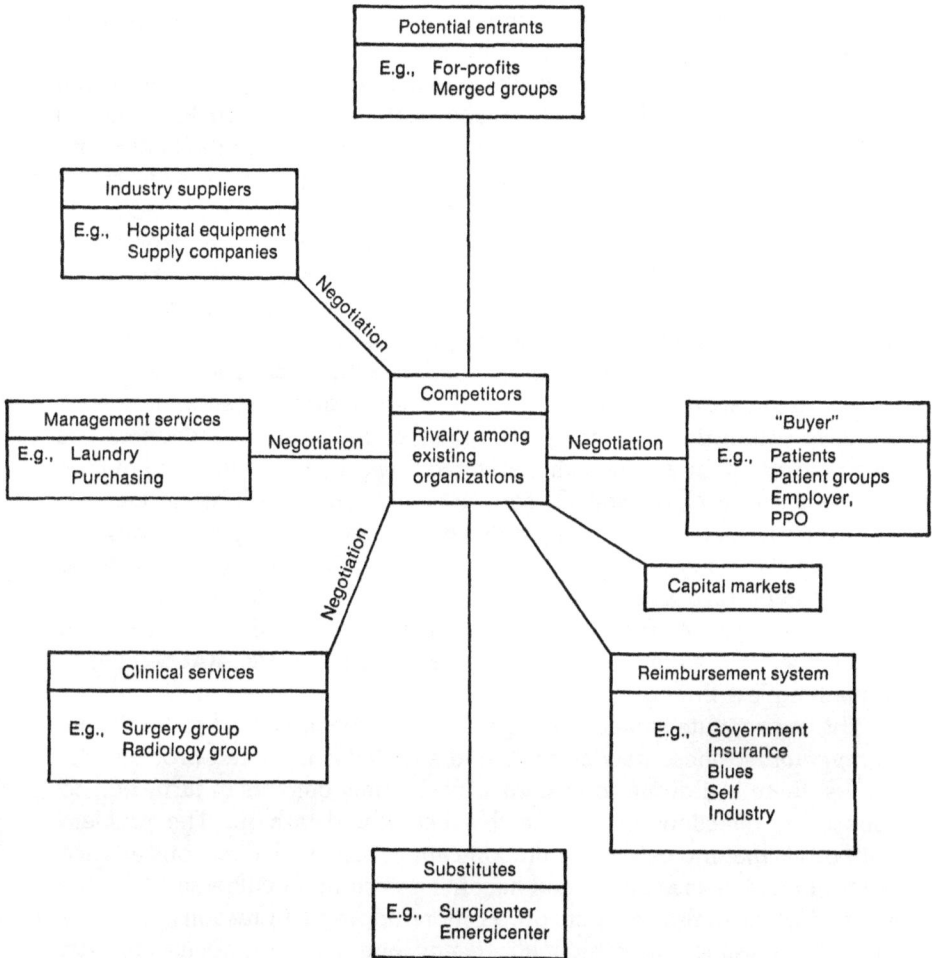

stitutions. One now-common responsive strategy is for hospitals to form a collaborative system which will have sufficient resources to combat potential new entrants. A more subtle, but more dangerous, new entrant is found in the non-patient-care sector. Many smaller hospitals experiencing problems seek managerial assistance from one of the many institutions now providing management services or management contracting. Often these are for-profit organizations. While the initial approach is in the management area, it is but a small step for patient-care referrals to begin to be redirected.

Traditionally, the health system consisted of hospitals which, for the most part, owned the array of health services existing in a particular area, i.e., ambulatory care and in-patient services. This hospital-based system was complemented by the individual practitioner. The past 20 years have seen the emergence of a wide array of free-standing patient-care services or *substitutes*, originating most often from non-hospital-based sources. A concern with the lack of care available to the poor led to the development of federally funded community health centers. A concern for reducing costs and providing preventive care led to the evolution of the HMO, and this, in turn, led to individual practitioners banding together to form the Independent Practice Association (IPA). The evolution of technology has led to the possibility of free-standing therapeutic or diagnostic clinics such as dialysis centers, cardiac evaluation centers, and surgicenters. Hospitals and industrial companies seeking new markets and new sources of revenue have seen gaps in the existing system or attractive market centers and have entered such segments as home health, where once the Visiting Nurse Associations (VNAs) held sway. In each instance, an area at least partially within the province of hospitals or individual practitioners has been picked off by a new entity, oriented toward a relatively small market segment with a highly specific service or product. The VNA in Denver, for example, had no competition five years ago. Now there are some 23 agencies providing various forms of home health care, few of which are as comprehensive as that of the VNA, but each of which is oriented towards some part of the market segment the VNA used to service. As a result, the VNA's market share has dropped from nearly 100 percent to something less than 60 percent.

The appropriate strategic response of organizations used to *traditional competitors* to these new entrants and substitutes is indeed problematic. At first there is a desire to face each of the new entrants in turn, i.e., to look in all directions in a somewhat bewildered fashion. The problem with this is that the existing institution cannot face in all directions at once without diluting its activities and becoming even more vulnerable to existing or further future competition. A more appropriate response is to review the existing organizational strategy and refine it, focusing upon those market segments most compatible with the distinctive competence of the organization and most attractive to the purposes of the organization, whether financial or social. A VNA such as the one in Denver cannot successfully compete with the total array of its competition. Should it, for example, get into the business of respite care, providing homemakers, or adult day centers? It might be reasonable for a Visiting Nurse Association to direct its attention more towards complex patients with higher-technology nursing needs. But again, the specific response has to be a function not only of an organization's competence but also of the existing or future reimbursement systems that will determine whether particular market segments are revenue producing or losing.

Traditionally, the health delivery industry has obtained medical equipment and supplies from a number of manufacturing and drug companies. These are what is termed *industry suppliers*. The relationship with suppliers has become increasingly complex in recent years. Much hospital equipment is now regulated by certificate of need (CON). To some degree, health delivery institutions may integrate backwards into supplying some of their own needs. Similarly, some hospital supply companies are getting into health delivery. More critical is the capacity of larger groups of health delivery institutions to negotiate a lower price with suppliers by joining together in joint purchasing and standardization. The development of computer-based inventory systems allows health delivery institutions to carry lower inventory and therefore work with lower operating capital. When one of the key regulatory forces is a demand for lower costs, the capacity of the health delivery organization to control its supply cost becomes critical.

It is now a truism to say that the situation of the *buyer* in the health care industry is far more complex than it is in traditional industry. For the most part, the patient as buyer does not purchase health care directly, that is, out-of-pocket. Most (but not all) patients are insured through one means or another, and for the most part, physicians determine what health services patients receive, often regardless of the patient's capacity to pay. So "buyers" may obtain health care, but the health delivery organization may get only part of the cost reimbursed. Payer mix and case mix are therefore important ways of measuring how much revenue a health organization gets for the mix of work it does. The situation is changing however, as more institutions get directly into marketing themselves. The nature of the reimbursement system will be discussed below as a separate competitive factor. Increasingly, efforts in health care organizations are directed towards groups of potential patients. Thus employers, concerned about benefits, seek to negotiate with HMOs or with hospitals that will reduce the employer's costs and provide employees with superior health care. This is now being done through the Preferred Provider Option (PPO) which gives a monopoly to the provider of choice. As competition in the health system heats up, health delivery organizations seek to secure sources of referral to ensure that their resources are fully utilized. Hospitals attempt, where possible, to secure a referral base through arrangements with a health maintenance organization (HMO), through employer contracts, or through the capture of primary care facilities which will send them patients to use their secondary and tertiary care resources. HMOs, in turn, seek contracts with employers and arrangements with hospitals.

But patients, and the physicians advising them, are not the only buyers. Thus, for example, the New England Medical Center Hospital in Boston, recognizing the need of HMOs for referral institutions, is attempting to develop a costing system that will make it the low-cost, high-quality provider of choice for HMOs in this area. This tactic is valuable in competing for HMO business. Here, the HMO is the buyer for the hospital's services.

With the evolving diagnosis-related group (DRG) reimbursement system (see below), hospitals can maximize income because they are paid for particular DRGs regardless of cost if the hospitals reduce their costs below their reimbursement level. The nature of the DRG system places a premium on having a "desirable" mix of patients, as some DRGs pay more than others. As a result, health institutions are paying much more attention to their patient mix, as well as beginning to segment their markets and address the different market segments more systematically with a varied range of services.

As the buyer becomes more powerful and more articulate about desired attributes, health delivery organizations are paying attention not only to better understanding the nature of their product or service, but also to designing particular products or services for particular market segments. An appendectomy is no longer simply an appendectomy. The Medical Center's strategy may be to provide a high-quality operation at the lowest cost if it is selling to an HMO. If it is attempting to reach "convenience" business, it may provide a different set of desirable attributes such as would be found in a surgicenter where the client, perhaps a busy businessperson, may get in and out rapidly, though not necessarily at as low a cost. A third possible product would be the "luxury" service that might be provided to the wealthy foreigner seeking comfortable accommodation at any price. Visiting Nurse Associations, dealing with their rapidly increasing competition, have traditionally analyzed their case load by patient visit, as though all patients were in a sense similar. Clearly, however, there are those patients requiring a single procedure once, and those patients requiring many complex procedures from a wide variety of professionals over a long period of time. These market segments require different kinds of resources, organized differently and marketed differently. Such patients also require a different kind of measurement if the market segments are to be understood properly. Patient complexity/episode, not patient visits, is now the basic unit of measurement.

As health delivery organizations recognize that they can no longer be all things to all people, they have to specialize and direct their resources economically; product market segmentation becomes a critical issue. Diagnostic and therapeutic procedures are not simple entities. It is the perceived benefits associated with various procedures that will determine whether or not those procedures are regarded as desirable purchases by the patient, employer, or physician. Marketing the quality of care as a set of attributes perceived to be desirable by the purchaser becomes important (Chapter 4). Thus, HMOs must compete for individual patients and patient groups (from employers) on the basis of cost, number, and quality of benefits.

In the past, *management services* were provided internally by the health delivery organization. They were therefore not considered supplied services. With both increased pressure to control costs and increased competition, however, health organizations have tended to move in one of two directions. Management services, once provided in-house by staff, may be contracted for so that the fixed costs associated with them diminish. Security services, for example, are often supplied under contract by an outside company. Similarly, laundry, rather than being done in-house, may be provided at lower cost by a laundry company. More recently, many health institutions have found themselves in the business of supplying management services, not only for themselves but for others, as a distinct business. Through restructuring and unbundling—separating activities once grouped together—institutions with excess capacity have seen an opportunity to develop some of their internal management services into a separate business. This not only reduces costs but also provides added sources of revenue. The development of such businesses is a form of strategic diversification. Management services may be contracted for or supplied to others as individual functions or as groups of functions. The latter is a currently popular direction called management contracting. Hospitals may secure a total range of management services from a management contracting company, or, if they possess excess capacity, may themselves provide the total range of management services to some smaller institution. While it does not necessarily pay in itself, management contracting often subsequently leads to the acquisition of smaller hospitals by a larger hospital providing management contract services.

Clinical services are an even more recent addition to the competitive array. Historically, most physicians have affiliated with one or more health institutions, usually several, on a fee-for-service basis. Health institutions have, in fact, little control over physicians, who may often work at several hospitals. With increased competition, this arrangement becomes more problematic, since physicians with numerous admitting privileges clearly have a choice as to which of several institutions they admit their patients. Any action on the part of a particular hospital may result in a physician transferring not only his skills but his patients to some other institution. This again illustrates the contradiction peculiar to health care: physicians not only supply services to an institution but also create patient demand; i.e., they are the marketing arm of the institution.

There have been two major trends recently. Hospitals, recognizing that they are vulnerable to the combined supply and demand aspects of physician services, have attempted to secure patients through direct marketing of their hospital services, as well as through developing contracts with groups of physicians to supply services on a negotiated basis. The trend towards physician groups is one that certainly benefits physicians and may benefit health institutions. The Robert Wood Johnson Foundation has funded the transformation of 15 medical clinics into medical group practices with the intent of enabling hospitals to obtain better control over costs, quality, and medical education.

The advantage to physicians of forming groups is fairly obvious. By banding together, the physicians can afford a greater degree of high-quality administrative services for themselves. Depending on whether they are a single specialty or multispecialty group, they can also provide some cross-referral within the group. Moreover, the combination of physicians constitutes a more powerful entity in negotiating with the institution. Hospitals also have some advantage, although they would probably prefer to deal with salaried physicians rather than contract with groups. With physician groups, as with unions, hospitals are dealing with a single entity, not diverse individuals. However, the failure to secure a contract with a particular group may mean the withdrawal of critical services and a significant volume of patients. Increasingly, some hospitals' chief executive officers regard physicians as essentially competition rather than an intrinsic part of the institution.

Capital markets are important as government funds for building dry up. Whether through bonds or venture capital, how can health organizations raise what they need and avoid exorbitant interest charges? Supergroups—groups of groups of hospitals—are sufficiently attractive that banks are becoming their partners. Lesser mortals can gain better bond ratings through associative collaboration of several institutions.

There has perhaps been as much change in the nature of *reimbursement systems* as in any other competitive factor in the health system. Instead of a cost-based system involving procedures or patient days, there is now a complex array of prospective systems with caps on revenue, or systems based upon various forms of diagnosis-related groups (DRGs). The intent of most new reimbursement systems is to minimize the rate of cost increases to the health system. Health organizations' strategies have altered accordingly. The nature of most DRG-based systems is to place an emphasis on having a "desirable" DRG case mix. Hospitals have therefore become far more aware of the nature of their case mix and of the importance of altering it in the direction of increased complexity, since reimbursement will be higher. Hospitals have also recognized the need to reduce costs and, for the first time, there is an advantage to holding costs down. In a cost-based system this was not true. Certain groups of patients were compensated for at a fixed level (e.g., Medicare patients) and could best be treated as a distinct market segment. Hospitals have even gone as far as providing services to the different segments through organizations distinct and separate from the remainder of the hospital. This has often been done through the process of restructuring and unbundling, the rationale being that a distinct corporation can allocate overhead in a way that is advantageous to the hospital.

Relevant Environment, Competitive Position, and Competitive Performance

Generally speaking, it is to a subset of the competitive forces that a health organization must primarily attend and toward which it addresses the major thrust of its strategy. New England Medical Center emphasizes being the low-cost/high-quality provider of choice among buyers. Hill Medical Center negotiates for a major grouping of regional institutions to compete with for-profits. Judgment is always, in essence, the sifting of forces in an effort to define the relevant environment, and thus, logically, what one plans to do.

Competitive position is a function of the relevant environment, and some useful measures are shown in Figure 2-4. Adaptive evaluation

Figure 2-4

Competitive Position

Number and diversity of markets/market segments
Number/size of competitors in markets/market segments
Growth/contraction of each market/market segment
Number of products in each market/market segment—self/competition
Market segment value—social and/or financial
Life-cycle stage of each product in each market/market segment for self/competition

takes a look at and measures how you are currently doing, how your position may be altering, and so how you will do in the future.

Middlesex County Hospital in Massachusetts had a virtual monopoly on tuberculosis care in its area, which was then well reimbursed. It therefore had a single product in a single market, with no competition, and more than broke even. Technology changed the buyer. Tuberculosis diminished, so the market shrank. The hospital decided to get into several distinct segments of the chronic/rehabilitation market—alcoholism, drug addiction, quadriplegia—by mixing custodial and restorative products and facing considerable competition. Moreover, the products were recent entries in a relatively mature market, and were poorly reimbursed at less than cost. It was not then surprising that trying so much in such financially questionable (though socially redeeming) areas resulted in a large deficit and political questions from the county government.

Competitive performance measures are quite distinct from many of the usual measures that health organizations find convenient. Bed occupancy rates and patient days or visits do not tell you much about how you are doing. Suggested measures are shown in Figure 2-5.

Figure 2-5

Competitive Performance

Share of market in each market/market segment
Growth in share
Growth rate in each market/market segment for each product/service
Market segment mix or product market value—proportion of favorable product market segments, e.g., payer and case mix
Perceived quality of product(s)
Quality/cost advantage
Quality/price advantage

It is quite possible, in a growing market, to do well without *increasing* share. However, whether an organization will benefit by share or growth depends on whether it is reimbursed for what it does (product/market value). Competitive advantage will be determined by how quality is perceived by the buyers and whether it is priced competitively (quality/price advantage) while still making money (quality/cost advantage) for the institution. Mature products for which the cost of innovation has been expended, are likely to have a quality cost advantage. Lest the reader feel this is all too pecuniary, it is salutary to remember that health institutions can only afford to give away care (as all probably should, to some degree, as long as there are the aging, indigent, and needy without the means to pay) if they can subsidize this care from some other source. HMOs recognize that to fulfill this aspect of their mission, they may need to seek special funding and not burden their competitive rates. Market-segment mix then becomes important, since one segment may be needed to subsidize another. But a diverse market-segment mix with many products/services in each segment requires a higher degree of organizational integration, which carries both financial and human cost.

The Relationship between Strategy, Business(es), State, and Performance

Adaptation means a fit between four factors: what is *needed* by the environment and the marketplace; what the environment and marketplace will *pay for;* the *strategy* of the organization; and how such strategy is addressed through the organization's internal resources, processes, and structure—its *state.* Strategy, through defining *mission, goals,* and *objectives,* sets up *tasks* which the state must carry out. Middlesex County

Hospital had a strategy of providing custodial care to chronic tuberculosis patients, a single simple task for which a simple organizational state sufficed. When the strategy changed, multiple, more complex tasks were added, requiring a complex organization.

Note that there may often be discrepancies between stated mission and actual strategy. The Cancer Care Cooperative of Western Massachusetts purported to provide *comprehensive* cancer care, but in its early days its member hospitals only gave *acute* care. Harvard Community Health Plan's mission intends to serve all socioeconomic strata and age groups. But early on it served primarily the middle class and young. More recently, it has altered strategy to fulfill its mission more broadly by placing centers in less affluent towns and by marketing to older age groups.

Note also that, in theory, structure follows strategy. In fact, the organization's state largely determines how it will perceive the relevant environment and, therefore, the strategic alternatives it is likely to consider and reject.

Evaluating adaptation means reconsidering your business strategy and state in the light of events. In practice, this may be less a conscious effort than a result of a series of positioning activities (see below). These activities may be precipitated by a worsening of competitive position, a series of moves set in motion by a subsystem, or a recognition that something must be done (though *what* is not yet clear). Positioning is akin to nudging a tanker into the right direction by the effort of tugs—the details of the course are not important at this point, but the direction is. You may know something is wrong, or at least not right, and have some sense of where you must not go and even vaguely of where you wish to go—but in the meantime, you can be preparing for the voyage by gaining a competitive positional advantage. To further the nautical metaphor, it is like getting a good jump over the starting line in a yacht race.

Clearly, if performance is off, or likely to be so as you project the future, then readaptation is needed. The extent to which this will require moving away from the historical state will tell you the level of resistance you may expect and the amount of change needed. A sense of general direction to harness positioning activities is important to avoid cross-purposes. This is the point where consultants can be of value since they do not share your staff's attachment to the past; they will not have the same blinkers on as they consider the future and redefine the relevant environment. An industrial example may be salutary. General Foods several years ago decided to review its strategy. Five of eight top managers felt initially that their growth goals could be achieved only if the existing strategy were well implemented. Consultants put the top management group through an intensive and extensive review of trends, strengths, weaknesses, etc. (as outlined here). After six months' work, all eight top managers agreed that the existing strategy could not succeed and must be altered. It was only then that they could be expected to review new alternative strategies dispassionately.

The key questions include: Are your goals and objectives still appropriate, even though you must change what you are doing to achieve them; or must you change your goals and objectives because they are no longer appropriate? Is your definition of your business(es) still appropriate? Have the tasks changed? If so, do you need to change your state to address those altered tasks? What must you change in your organizational state? These questions form the subject of the next part of this chapter. The redefinition of your business(es) is a delicate problem, especially when you are used to and value the past definition. Is an HMO in the HMO business or in the prepaid health care business? The definition determines the relevant competitive factors and therefore the relevant environments. If it wishes to grow nationally, it could set up or acquire other HMOs. Or it could develop hybrid arrangements with already existing Independent Practice Associations (IPAs) which have lower capital requirements, and thus reduce local resistance and the cost of expansion. It could even redefine its business(es) along three dimensions and be in the insurance business (providing to consumers integrated packages of insurance covering home, health, and life), the prevention business (providing programs of diagnosis, exercise, and diet), as well as the health care business (providing primary care and referral, linked to the insurance through prepaid premiums). This strategy—with its radically different definition of the "business(es)"—would require very different organizational states in each business.

Organizational State

As with strategic planning, every author has an array of organizational state variables that he or she regards as important and displays in different ways.[9-11] In essence, however, all look at much the same things, and Figure 2-6 represents a synthesis based on the work of a variety of authors.

What really is an organizational state? What governs how the outside world is perceived, and what must be changed when that outside world gets out of synch with the inside world? These questions are answered below.

---

[9]Ibid.

[10]Quinn, *Strategies for Change.*

[11]*Business Policy.*

Figure 2-6

Organizational State

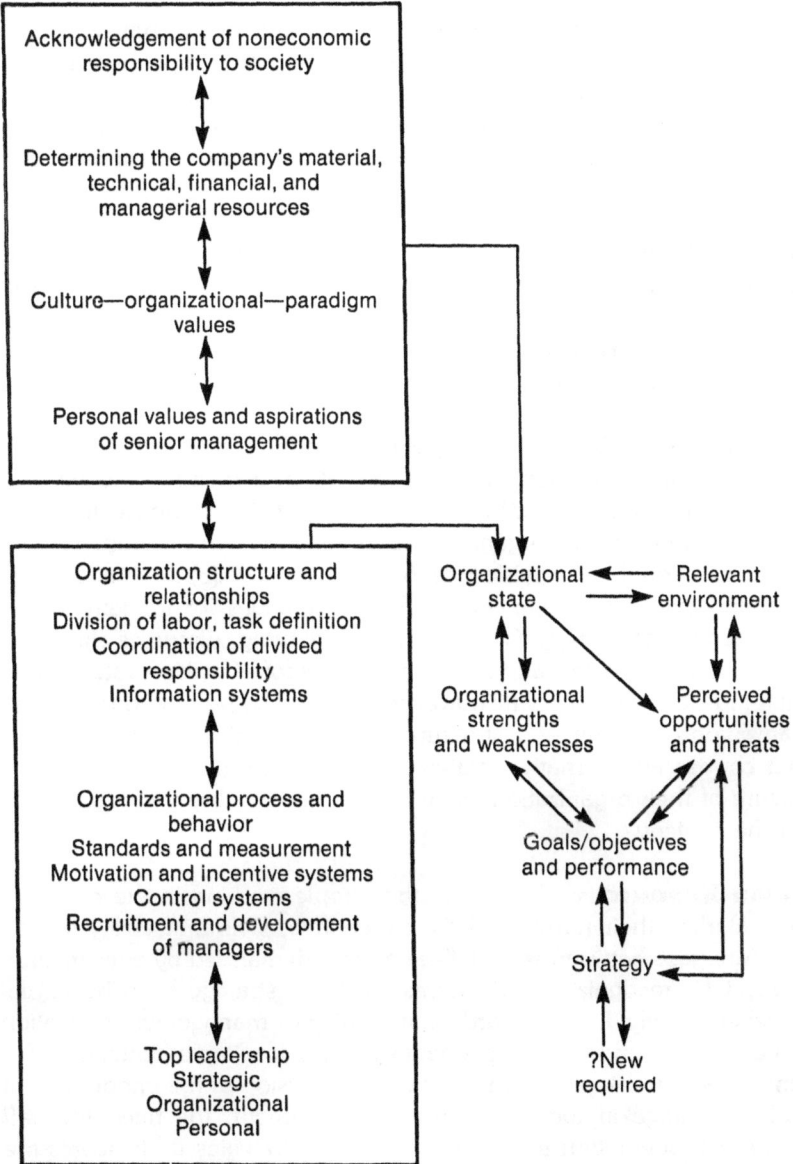

| Acknowledgement of noneconomic responsibility to society |
| Determining the company's material, technical, financial, and managerial resources |
| Culture—organizational—paradigm values |
| Personal values and aspirations of senior management |

Organization structure and relationships
Division of labor, task definition
Coordination of divided responsibility
Information systems

Organizational process and behavior
Standards and measurement
Motivation and incentive systems
Control systems
Recruitment and development of managers

Top leadership
Strategic
Organizational
Personal

Organizational state → Relevant environment

Organizational strengths and weaknesses

Perceived opportunities and threats

Goals/objectives and performance

Strategy

?New required

Organizational Strengths and Weaknesses   These comprise a profile of assets and skills of the organization relative to those of its competitors.

Personal Values of Managers   These refer to the motivations and needs of the key executives who must develop and implement strategy. Again, these values and motivations may be based on the current paradigm. Managers may thus find the need for a paradigm change which supports new motives, incentives, and strategies more appropriate to the current environment.

Organizational Opportunities and Threats   These define perception of the relevant environment with its attendant risks and rewards.

Societal Expectations   These reflect the impact of government policy, consumer desires, evolving mores, etc. on health care organizations.

Organizational Structure   This refers to the formal authority hierarchy and reporting structure of the organization. Structure describes how an organization focuses staff efforts on particular tasks and relationships. In general, three major organizational structures have evolved: (1) centralized functional, (2) division or service oriented (3) matrix. Each of these structures has advantages and disadvantages for implementing a particular type of strategy. Chapter 6, Restructuring, discusses alternative organizational structures and their implications for effective strategy in the health industry. At this point, however, it should be pointed out that if an organization's strategy and structure are incompatible, managers must either choose an alternative strategy which will work within the existing structure of their organization or be ready to restructure the organization to fit the strategy.

Human Resources   These are the people working in the organization, including their number, skills, experience, style and ability to perform. Any gaps between staff skills and tasks demanded by a given strategy must be recognized and addressed if the strategy is to be implemented effectively. In this regard, staff training or management education can become essentially complementary tasks for implementation of a given strategy. In keeping with our earlier discussion of the importance of paradigm change in today's turbulent environment, the need for staff training or reorientation to implement certain strategies underscores the relationship between strategy, change in organizational behavior, and change in staff attitudes and skills. These may be short term or long term and require the development of new *types* of skills.

Culture This is "informal organization" and is best seen as how things are really done in an organization. This element is also closely related to the notion of a paradigm as a tool in the strategy implementation process. Culture is tied closely to an organization's history and, like the broader societal concept of culture, refers to a perspective which is shared by those in a particular group. Culture is comprised of those conventional behaviors and understandings that characterize societies. It is passed on, evolves slowly, and is difficult to change. Understanding what works well in an organizational culture will encourage the development of strategic decisions that produce exceptional results. Again, however, where there is conflict between organizational culture and strategic choice, managers may face the need to change strategy or change "culture." To support a long-term strategy which is based on major changes in organizational behavior, some fundamental change in internal culture may be necessary.

Organizational and Management Processes These refer to the systems used to keep an organization moving towards its strategic objectives. Such processes usually include planning, programming, budgeting, and personnel incentives.

In toto, this model illustrates not only the organizational elements which should determine strategic choice, but also the elements which will affect implementation of strategic choices. Effective strategies begin and are formulated within a context that takes stock of both the organization's internal state and its external environment. Whether a selected strategy can be implemented must also be assessed within that double context. Any internal changes which are dictated by the strategy (in systems, staff, culture, or structure) should be explicitly designed to drive the organization towards its chosen strategic objectives.

Life is the art of drawing sufficient conclusions from insufficient premises.

Samuel Butler

Positioning

Porter believes that an effective competitive strategy involves offensive or defensive action to create a defendable position against competitive forces.[12] This broadly involves a number of possible approaches:

---

[12]Porter, *Competitive Strategy.*

Positioning the organization so that its capabilities provide the best defense against the existing array of competitive forces.

Influencing the balance of forces through strategic moves, thereby improving the organization's relative position.

Anticipating shifts in the factors underlying the forces and responding to them, thereby exploiting change by choosing a strategy appropriate to the new competitive balance before rivals recognize it.

Porter goes on to describe positioning as an attempt to build defenses against competitive forces or as seeking a position where the forces are weakest. Influencing the balance is an offensive strategy which does not merely cope but is meant to alter causes.

As health delivery organizations seek to contend with the competitive forces discussed above, they not only determine the need for change in direction, but may also begin to take strategic actions, i.e., engage in positioning activities that secure an advantageous competitive position, moving the organizations generally in the strategic direction they plan to follow. Positioning activities are then both preparation for strategy and at the same time the beginning of its implementation. But implementation of a strategy often involves more profound changes in organizational state than those required to position (see below). Positioning can take place regardless of whether a final strategy has been articulated or not; though as stated above, the activities require a sense of direction (i.e., does the positioning activity move you toward or away from a desired competitive position?) and the activities must be consonant with one another (i.e., not in conflict with each other or with the evolving strategy).

Positioning therefore enables managers to place their organization so that its capabilities provide the best competition against other organizations, influence the balance of forces to improve the organization's relative position, and give the organization the greatest possible flexibility to respond to any anticipated shifts in competitive forces. Taking advantage of options requires lead time, or they disappear; so positioning may need to occur well in advance (five years!) of a potentially worsening competitive situation. This is why such activities may be controversial; the situation requiring them may only be obvious to top management, with its longer time perspective.

The model includes five major positioning activities:

Scanning.
Product/market analysis.
Collaboration.
Restructuring.
Managing the physician.

These topics are dealt with individually in subsequent chapters of this book, so each will be discussed only briefly below.

Positioning activities are required if an organization is going to be able to implement a successful competitive strategy, given the complex and uncertain environment in which health care organizations now function. Basically, in positioning itself for strategic activities, each health delivery organization addresses and responds to the subset of particular competitive forces, i.e., the relevant environment which it regards as most significant for its own competitive situation. It is important to reemphasize that an assessment of the salience of the competitive forces is an absolute prerequisite to considering how any health organization should position itself. Thus, for example, if it is felt that the major competitive threat is from a change in the reimbursement system, a hospital, for example, may feel that it has to address its patient mix and improve the mix through product/market analysis and restructuring. Another hospital, less threatened because it has a favorable DRG mix, may recognize that its major competitive threat comes from new entrants in its market area.

All positioning activities are intended to reduce information uncertainty and increase resource availability, and thus make more certain the future success of competitive strategy which is always, remember, a judgment of an uncertain future situation.

Scanning

In an era of complexity and environmental uncertainty, the ability to adapt to the environment as it changes in unpredictable ways becomes critical to the health care organization. Not only must senior management project changes so that it can institute appropriate strategic decisions in a proactive fashion; managers must also attempt to influence the environment where that is possible. The scanning and tracking function must be done internally and externally. The fact that many health care organizations are small and unable to afford a corporate planning capacity means that they may have to rely on external sources for this function. Increasingly, one value of collaborative endeavors is that they provide a resource capacity that can absorb a corporate planning function. As health care organizations seek to extend their activities and consider diversified business, they must be aware of strategic opportunities and have the capacity to do feasibility studies to determine whether these opportunities should and could be taken advantage of. In an era of less complexity and change, this function could easily be performed by top management. This is no longer true. Internal tracking of performance is also crucial for obvious reasons.

Product Market Analysis

One way of reducing uncertainty is for a health delivery organization to understand better exactly what it offers. The ultimate strategy may be to offer a range of products/services to a range of market segments, or it may be to restrict offerings to a narrowed range. For example, as Midland Hospital, a small, acute care facility, considers its future, it is in a three-way competition with two larger hospitals. At best, without initiating change, the hospital will be left to address itself to those aspects of health care unwanted by its two larger competitors. If Midland wishes to enter favorable areas of activity, it will need a more powerful position than it occupies at present. For this hospital, product market analysis leads inevitably to the conclusion that Midland must position itself through collaboration to be able to choose from a wider set of options and not have to settle for a residual role.

The Maria Nursing Home is faced with an even more difficult problem. This nursing home, while quite successful, does not provide enough revenue to support its aging order of founding nuns. The home must move into some new market segment to provide additional revenues. But which? Only product market analysis can provide an answer.

The Visiting Nurse Association of Denver, once providing the range of services required by clients at home, faces increasing competition. Should it continue to supply this range of services or should it narrow its offering to specific market segments?

Beyond understanding product market segmentation, an issue which will be addressed in a later chapter, is the contentious issue of the possibility of marketing quality of care. Economists addressing the quality issue point out that consumers in health care generally tend to be disappointed with quality. Performance is often uneven and unpredictable as services expand, so average quality drops and disappointment arises.[13] Whatever the objective attributes of quality, which tend to be associated with the technical dimensions of care rather than the humanistic ones, quality essentially has to do with what people want versus what they receive. It is possible in health care, as in other areas of market research, to determine the attributes that the consumer wants or values. Efforts can then be made to supply those attributes either to the experienced consumer or, with greater difficulty, to the inexperienced or naive consumer.

Collaboration

The benefits of collaboration are essentially securing additional resources or additional markets (or share of market) through some form of

---

[13] A. O. Hirschman, *Shifting Involvement: Private Interest and Public Action* (Princeton, N.J.: Princeton University Press, 1982).

association. Too often, however, health care institutions talk collaboration without any real understanding of the ends that are desirable. Collaboration should always be directed towards some end. Collaboration may take a variety of forms. Chapter 5 will discuss the key factors indicating whether collaboration is desirable in terms of whether organizations are complementary and matching organizational styles. Given the relatively small size of most health care delivery organizations, it is not surprising that many seek to augment resources or markets through this means. A final point that will be repeated: Most health institutions compete and collaborate with others simultaneously; therefore, the collaborative structure must be able to accommodate this basic ambivalence or it will fail.

Restructuring

The fourth positioning activity is restructuring. As health delivery organizations review the competitive forces and determine individual, desired strategies, they must also review the extent to which their existing organization is being strained and/or will allow them to move in their desired direction. Can resources, perhaps gained through collaboration, be better allocated through reshaping at the organizational and/or corporate level? When and how an organization should restructure, and what activities might be unbundled into new organizations which can take advantage of new possibilities without constraint will be addressed in Chapter 6.

Managing the Physician

Physicians traditionally dominated health care institutions. As managerial competence has assumed greater importance, one might (erroneously) draw the conclusion that in some instances physicians have become an unpalatable fact of life. However, physicians still remain critical as resources and marketers. As the interests of institutions and physicians diverge, the nature of the relationship between physician and organization becomes ever harder to manage. This issue will be covered more fully in Chapter 7. For now, the key issues can be boiled down to two. The first is the extent to which the physician should be involved in the direction of the institution as it moves to ever more diversified activities, on the one hand. And the second is the way in which physician activities can be directed toward the interests of the institution through the design of appropriate incentives, on the other. While physicians are the primary focus, other professionals, e.g., nurses, are also critically important, especially since task shifting (e.g., from physicians to nurse practitioners) often means cost savings. But again, one can expect inertia as traditional roles, values, and incentives constrain adoption of innovative problem solutions.

Competitive Strategies

Goldsmith, in a book on hospital survival, describes three strategies for hospitals: horizontal integration (hospital groups); vertical integration (the capture of referral sources); and the management of physician-hospital relationships.[14] The Harvard Business School teaches a different version.[15]

Competitive strategy is oriented to the set of competitive forces identified as significant to an institution. The *particular* form it will take is a function of the type of institution (hospital group, VNA) and the particular circumstances. The general categories fall within two dimensions:

High growth	Maintenance
on site	Focus
off site	Differentiation
Low growth	Diversification
	Mini-health-system (vertical integration)

These are not mutually exclusive within either dimension since a hospital group, for instance, can grow fast in certain areas and slowly in others, or engage both in diversification and differentiation. A hospital may maintain certain product markets and focus investment on others. If it regards the reimbursement system as key, it may differentiate itself as the low-cost provider for selected DRGs.

No-growth strategies are no longer viable options in today's environment. Managers should accept the fact that for any type of health care organization today, it is no longer possible simply to stand still. The escalation of costs and the degree of competition mean that even the organization which does not wish to become more complex or to grow as a strategic option has, in fact, to grow to some degree to stay where it is.

Maintenance

This corresponds to the "no-change" strategy—the past pattern of activities continues. It can continue at a higher level of investment if high growth is desired, and at the original site or through the acquisition of like institutions collaborating associatively.

Focus

Focus on limited special opportunity is a strategy that tends to be well regarded by organizations that have started out in a focused fashion, but

---

[14]J. C. Goldsmith, *Can Hospitals Survive? The New Competitive Health Care Market* (Homewood, Ill.: Dow Jones-Irwin, 1981).

[15]*Business Policy.*

poorly regarded by those that have had a broad base of activity. Thus, a free-standing ambulatory care center may have no difficulty in continuing this focused life. A small, acute care general hospital may find it difficult to consider contracting its activities and limiting itself to long-term or ambulatory care. Yet many small, acute care hospitals are facing exactly these options. Those that embrace them aggressively may well have an active, successful, and exciting future life.

Focus means narrowing the current mix of activities or efforts, but can also mean increasing the volume of activities within this mix. Within a focus strategy there are low-growth and high-growth options. Could Midland make a focus strategy work? Probably not as a sole entity, since it is unlikely that a small, 250-bed, acute care hospital can continue to exist in a three-way competition with two large hospitals unless it focuses on residual areas, such as long-term and psychiatric care, which would be unacceptable to its medical staff. Preserving its options requires that it collaborate and thus retain some power over *what* it focuses on. An example of a high-growth focus strategy might be a small, previously acute care general hospital which decides to emphasize teenage care and geriatric care and builds several centers to deliver this to a broader market than that served by the original hospital. Roman Catholic systems such as the Health Corporation of the Archdiocese of Newark or the Medical Center of Queens and Brooklyn, New York, could focus upon the provision of health care to Catholic populations. But the demographic mix of their immediate communities is such that Catholics would not necessarily constitute the majority of their patients. Again, this would be a risky strategy.

Focus is therefore possible only when market share can be maintained or increased by limiting patient care activities and/or targeting selected patient populations. Focus is also an appropriate strategy for an organization which provides a highly specialized service, such as dialysis. It is also particularly suited to very narrow market segments where the organization achieves its goals by better meeting particular needs and/or meeting service needs at a lower cost.

Differentiation

Differentiation involves creating something that is perceived as being unique. Harvard Community Health Plan (HCHP) has managed successfully to differentiate its central city HMO centers from those of others by emphasizing particular attributes, including the Harvard name, high quality, and moderate cost which appeal to the relatively mobile, highly sophisticated market. This strategy may be eroded as new HMOs compete on quality and cost. Moreover, the "brand" image, associated with academic excellence and technical quality, could be a drawback in a blue-collar town concerned more with community responsiveness.

Cleveland Clinic differentiates itself from other clinics through its proven high-technology capacity. South Clinic, on the other hand, once was differentiated on the dimension of superb humanistic patient care, but more recently the clinic has found its differentiated position eroded by the evolution of larger community hospitals and the movement of other institutions into this market segment (Chapter 8).

Diversification

Allowable patient-care cost and revenues are increasingly becoming limited through the placement of caps. The response on the part of health care providers is to seek alternate sources of income, either from patient-care revenues not subject to caps, or from other kinds of business altogether. Essentially there are three strategic responses to reimbursement limits. The first seeks to unbundle new types of patient-care revenue through the creation of separate corporations not subject to regulation. A later chapter on restructuring lists a number of efforts by major organizations in this regard. American Medical International, for example, has formed separate corporations to do cardiopulmonary function testing, respiratory therapy services, and physical therapy.

A second approach is to spin off management services, taking them out of the hospital and into a separate corporation where they, too, may not be subject to regulation. These services can then be sold back to the institution or to other clients. Many examples are given in the restructuring chapter, the most popular being the provision of shared services, for example, laundry and purchasing through a shared services corporation. Generally speaking, these management services are still allied to the health industry and the services required by it. Third, some health care organizations, recognizing the need for revenue, are getting into areas of business even further afield. These organizations form corporations which, while they may manage, for example, the real estate of the institution, may also put up parking lots or even own shopping centers. The essential purpose of the strategic option of diversifying business is to create new sources of revenue.

These strategies obviously have implications not only for organizational structure (the new types of organizations must be protected from regulatory constraints by being spun off into new corporations), but also for the type of management required to run these new enterprises successfully. As in new businesses anywhere, diversified business requires entrepreneurial managers who are given a great deal of freedom and latitude to pursue growth aggressively. It should be recognized that any health delivery organization entertaining the strategic option of moving into diversified business must consider the potential strain between its traditional management style and that required by the strategic option.

The Mini-Health-System

The mini-health-system is what is known in the industrial literature as vertical integration. Vertical integration is essentially an attempt to capture and control the sources of supply (by vertical integration backwards) and the outputs (by forward integration). Thus, a major publishing company might seek to integrate backwards by purchasing timberland and printing companies, and to integrate forward by acquiring retail bookstores. The equivalent in the health care field might be for a hospital to control the sources of supply of patients (ambulatory care or HMOs), as well as the sources of care after patients leave hospitals, e.g., nursing homes or home health agencies.

Such a strategy does not necessarily have to be geographically based. For example, major referral institutions such as Baylor in Texas are seeking to secure sources that supply tertiary care patients from countries as far away as Saudi Arabia. This is done through arrangements with local hospitals whereby Baylor provides management contracting services to the hospitals in return for referral. Generally speaking, however, the mini-health-system option is geographically based. Increasingly, hospital groups, formed through some form of collaboration, extend into the acquisition or development of primary care centers on the one hand, and nursing homes and long-term care on the other. Such mini-health-systems may be solely owned or, more commonly, formed through looser collaborative relationships. The essential purpose is to capture and retain the flow of patients within the system. Nursing Homes Associated (NHA) does this for the over-65 market through the provision of a total range of services: physical assessment, nursing home care at all levels, old age homes, and day-care centers, in one large city. Since many types of organizations are extending their range through this strategy, mini-health-systems arise from very different origins.

Conclusion

While maintenance, focus, differentiation, diversified business, and the mini-health-system are the major strategic options available for health delivery organizations in an era of uncertainty, few, if any, individual institutions or organizational groups will adopt a single, pure strategy. For the most part, some mix is appropriate and is what will be seen in practice.

Chapter 8 develops this in more detail, but some typical strategies used by a variety of institutions may be briefly considered here. Maria Nursing Home is a small nursing home run by an order of nuns now requiring additional revenues beyond the capacity of its existing size. A focus/growth strategy is unlikely to be successful because of regulations and market limitations. Moreover, limitations on the home's capacity to raise capital and on management's capacity make it impossible to consider major moves. The most likely option is for the home to move into some diversified business in an area closely allied with the existing one. Environmental analysis may reveal the need for other types of care for the elderly such as the provision of respite centers, old age homes, protected apartments, etc. These would not represent businesses sufficiently different to create a strain or a major demand upon capital.

The Harvard Community Health Plan (HCHP) has pursued a differentiated growth strategy. It has grown by design from one center in 1969 to five at present. As it has grown, it has also moved somewhat into a mini-health-system strategy springing from the need to acquire its own hospital for referral purposes rather than relying solely upon contractual arrangements. Changes in the environment are now putting pressure upon this strategy. Fourteen HMOs now exist in the greater Boston area, while employer enrollments are slackening with the recession. Hospital use and hospitalization costs have also risen faster than estimated. HCHP now faces questions about whether its growth goal continues to be realistic and whether the goal can be attained through the existing strategy, one which essentially assumes that the nature of HCHP's business is the HMO, i.e., prepaid preventive health care provided through discrete centers. Actually, the HMO business consists of three separate elements, each of which might represent a distinct business: (1) an emphasis on prevention; (2) the provision of prepaid health care; and (3) the provision of prepaid health care through discrete centers. Independent Practice Associations (IPAs) such as Doctor's Health Service, compete in the same prepaid market but with a different strategy, that of providing prepaid care through physician's offices. Could HCHP consider moving into the IPA business? Should it consider the possibility of providing prepaid health care directly to employers on industrial sites? May the specific needs of local communities conflict with the HCHP brand image? And finally, are "general purpose" centers the appropriate distribution mechanism for implementation? Is it more efficient, for example, to have various specialists doing daily sessions at each HCHP center or to have them grouped in a specialized diagnostic and referral center conveniently placed some distance from a series of primary care centers?

The Health Corporation of the Archdiocese of Newark (HCAN), a hospital group consisting of one teaching hospital and two smaller community hospitals, faces a number of strategic questions. It is clear that they need to enter into some diversified business to provide additional sources of revenue in an environment that is both economically constrained and highly competitive. But more critically, should HCAN pursue a differentiated strategy or a mini-health-system strategy? In other words, the choice is between operating an integrated system, perhaps acquiring additional primary care centers and long-term care facilities, or providing minimal corporate guidance to three separate institutions, each competing independently in its own market segments. A similar Roman Catholic hospital group, the Catholic Health Association of Brooklyn and Queens, has clearly chosen to go heavily into diversified business by withdrawing many of the management services from its member hospitals and creating a central corporate structure that now involves over 700 people. This central capacity currently provides management services to each member hospital and is poised to provide similar services to a wider range of clients.

The critical issue in chosing between strategic options is to determine realistic goals that reflect, on the one hand, the needs of a market and, on the other, the values of those running the institution. The definition and redefinition of relevant environments is crucial. Moreover, within the context of relevant environments, managers must continually reassess the business that they are in. A careful specification of organizational goals and an essential mission are critical to addressing these issues.

Summary

Strategy is not generally, in real life, first conceptualized, then implemented. Managers act to improve the competitive position of the organization and then articulate strategy.

Organizations are well adapted if their strategy is properly directed to their competitive position and they are well organized. A poorly adapted organization will perform poorly because it has an incorrect strategy or is not properly organized to implement that strategy. Organizations must change strategy if their competitive position alters.

The competitive model is intended to lay out how an organization's managers should assess their situation and alter what they do.

The environmental trends (demographic, economic, technological, regulatory, political and legal, social, and lifestyle) must be assessed as they alter and affect competitive forces.

The competitive forces must be assessed, as they will influence competitive position. The forces include traditional competition, new competition, competitive substitutes, capital markets, reimbursement systems, the buyer, industrial suppliers, administrative services, and clinical services. Managers regard a subset of these forces as significant and direct their activities and strategies towards this relevant environment. Information coming from outside of the relevant environment may often be ignored, even though it may be important. Managers must redefine their relevant environments from time to time.

Competitive position must be assessed. This includes looking at the number of markets that the organization is in; how many competitors there are in each market; and how these markets are growing; how many products (or services) there are in each market; what the life-cycle of each is; and finally, what the market segment value is both in financial and social terms.

Managers then determine goals, objectives, and strategy. They organize to harness resources towards those ends. While organizational structure should follow strategy, in practice, the way that an organization is structured often determines what it looks at and therefore what it regards as possible to do.

Finally, the organization assesses competitive performance, looking at share of market, growth of share, absolute growth, perceived quality, quality cost advantage, quality price advantage, and product market value.

Managers look ahead to determine whether, even if in the past the organization was well adapted, trends and competitive forces will influence future competitive position so that performance will be adversely affected. If so, managers need to reconsider what they are doing. They may need to redefine the business(es) that they are in. They may need to engage in positioning activities intended to improve competitive position. Positioning activities must not be at cross-purposes one with another.

Positioning activities include: scanning, the assessment of outside forces affecting the organization, and internal structure and performance. Product market analysis involves understanding the products that the organization is providing to the markets that it is interested in. The technical and human aspects of quality (and costs) are quite different. Competition in health care increasingly will involve quality and cost trade-offs. Collaboration allows entering markets or aggregating resources. The activities that require collaboration and whether or not there is a fit between organizations and processes of collaboration are crucial. Restructuring is the reconsideration of how resources are directed toward strategic ends. Managing the physician is critical to making strategies work. Hospitals must manage costs, productivity, and case mix if they are to be successful, and these are controlled by physicians who, in turn, must be better managed than they are now.

After positioning activities, strategy may be articulated and, if required, redirected. Basic strategies are: maintenance, the continuation of the previous set of activities; and focus, a narrowing of a set of activities. Diversification adds kinds of business for essentially financial reasons; differentiation distinguishes the set of activities of the organization from others by emphasizing critical characteristics; the mini-health-system (vertical integration) adds to the range of health care activities to more successfully capture patients.

If strategy is redirected, changes in the organization will be necessary, and these may be extensive and difficult to implement, requiring special techniques.

Adaptation, then, involves assessing trends and forces, determining the relevant environment, and defining goals, objectives, and strategy addressed to that environment. Readaptation involves redefining the business, engaging in positioning activities, redirecting strategy, and changing the organization.

Scanning

Two men look out through the same bars.
One sees mud, and one sees stars.
Frederick Lanbridge

In the previous chapter, the concept of *positioning* was introduced. *Scanning* refers to the process by which managers should gather information and analyze their organization's competitive position. In this regard, some scanning activities must precede and monitor other positioning activities. For example, an institution must scan its market area to determine what section of that market it wishes to serve before positioning itself either to develop a more specialized set of services for a narrowly defined market segment or to broaden its activities to compete against other agencies in the area. Scanning activities also provide a feedback loop to managers on how well their organizations are responding to the implementation of other positioning activities. For example, restructuring (Chapter 6) may be one positioning activity which a hospital undertakes to implement a longer-range competitive strategy. Scanning may reveal, however, that in the process of restructuring, the hospital is thwarting its efforts in other service areas deemed valuable and desirable to its mission. Based on this feedback, a manager may decide to revise the initial strategy and adopt one that will not require fundamental restructuring. In this case, scanning provides an intermediate monitoring function which leads to strategy re-formulation.

Scanning is an "inside-outside" activity vis-à-vis positioning: on the one hand, scanning precedes and drives other positioning activities. On the other, scanning is, itself, a fundamental positioning activity which must be done in conjunction with, or even subsequent to, others.

Benefits of Scanning

The competitive strength of an organization is critically bound up with the acquisition and analysis of information which promotes managers' abilities to create strategic options. The information obtained by scanning—about the environment, the organization, competitors, consumers, and success or failure in adapting effectively to the environment—provides the basis on which managers create and assess alternative strategic options.

In the past, health care organizations have shown a marked propensity to remain closed systems, limiting the quantity and variety of information which they take in and incorporate in their decision-making processes. Scanning, however, intrinsically refers to an organization's "looking outward." Managers of organizations must study their environments, assessing the many factors which were discussed in detail in Chapters 1 and 2; they must also study their organization's past experiences in addressing the environment, and change behavior in such a way that the organizations can adapt proactively to environmental changes. Initially, it is critical to take in large amounts of information to accurately identify and evaluate strategic options. (This process is visualized in Figure 3-1.) In the final analysis, however, managers must narrow their information intake while critical strategic decisions are actually being made. Of course, managers differ in their capacity to handle uncertainty. Some will want to gather more information for a longer time, before closing off to make a decision. This can be a source of problems in an organization if top managers differ among themselves in this regard. But a decision cannot be made while information is still being gathered which can alter that decision. Once the scan is completed, the utility of good scanning is that the organization may be able to change in ways that the manager wishes (proactively), rather than being forced to change in ways that management may not have chosen had it had the time, foresight, and information to be proactive.

A man must make his opportunity as oft as he finds it.
Francis Bacon

Figure 3 - 1

Preparation for Strategy Formulation

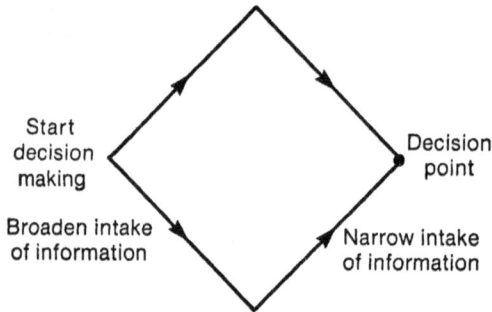

Who Should Scan?

All organizations should scan, and should do so on a regular basis, with additional, periodic, intensive scans every three to five years to capture any major changes in the environment, sociopolitical and economic trends, or regulatory policies. Organizations should also project trends for three- to five-year intervals based on current data. The latter encourages managers to remain proactive and forward thinking. Many organizations, however, do not have the internal staff to gain and interpret the information generated by scanning. In this era of environmental complexity and uncertainty, it is important that managers either develop this capacity in-house or rely on consultant staff to collect and interpret such information. For organizations which already have the in-house capability to scan and interpret the data from a scan, thought should be given to upgrading this capacity—possibly by increasing the amount of resources allocated to this corporate function.

But linking the scanning function—whether corporate, consulting, or computerized—to managerial decision making is absolutely crucial. Corporate planners are too often out of touch with managerial realities, or even worse, information is ignored when it signals danger because the function is not properly linked. Managers should plan with the help of planners, not the other way around.

To be balanced, scanning should be both internal and external to the organization. That is, managers need information on the internal operations of their organization as well as on the external environments. A recent article in *Fortune* magazine makes the point that more is required to improve corporate performance than understanding "a few simple [strategic] rules" based on external facts.[1] Scanning must also provide data on the organization itself and its capacity to adopt certain types of strategy.

Strategic management requires an interactive, unified process of strategy formulation and implementation. As has been argued, however, this should not be viewed as two distinct steps. Right from the beginning, strategic issues arising in any organization should be viewed in the broad context of implementation. Isolated from the realities of the organization's particular structure, systems, staff, and culture, strategies that appear sound in the abstract may simply not work. Scanning provides the preliminary data that suggests which strategies may and may not work in the context of an organization; equally important, it provides intermediate information on the effects of changes in organizational behavior and/or processes initiated in moving towards a strategy. Scanning activities also provide the information needed to monitor the interplay between various positioning activities, initial strategic objectives, and the possible need to articulate a revised strategy or to engage in additional positioning activities. As the staff of MAC, a well-known management consulting group, point out, resolving the internal strategic problems that beset one area of an organization requires a broad informational base.[2] An organization's various parts cannot be separated. Changing the incentive structure for physicians, for example, cannot be accomplished without a clear understanding of the attitudes of physicians, how their tasks and interrelationships with the organization are structured, and what is valued about their role in the culture of the organization. To make changes in a vacuum is very likely to produce disappointing results. A balance must be maintained between all the elements of a strategy, and scanning provides the information for this purpose.

Information for Scanning

All health care institutions maintain certain types of data on a regular basis which support their in-house functions. However, the key difference between the regular service/operation data maintained by most organizations and the information produced by scanning is the element of strategy. In other words, when you engage in scanning you seek information which can be used to answer specific strategic questions: Where are our strengths and weaknesses? What is this institution's "product"? Who con-

---

[1]"Corporate Strategists Under Fire," *Fortune*, 27 December 1982, pp. 15-20.

[2]P. Stonich, ed., *Implementing Strategy: Making Strategy Happen* (New York: Ballinger Publishing, 1982), p. 20.

stitutes (what types of patients) our primary service market? Our competitors' markets? Notably, this may require that managers (or planners engaged in scanning) use different approaches in measuring and presenting information, e.g., defining a "product cost" versus charges per admission, or collecting data from diagnosis-related groups (DRGs). This is, of course, desirable because in the process of determining what information they need, and in what forms, managers must cast their informational needs and interests in strategic terms.

Throughout, this book presents the spectrum of different types of information managers will need for positioning activities. Figure 3-2 outlines a functional process by which these data might be compiled.

Compiling data for positioning activities will require hard work, especially if there is no precedent for scanning in an organization. To be effective, there should be some organized mechanism to ensure that the process is efficient. The elements of this system can vary according to the particular organization's strategic needs and its staff capability. In some organizations, scanning functions might be performed effectively by one person, but this will likely be the exception rather than the rule. There are numerous sources for information—both published and unpublished—and many individuals in the organization can contribute to the information-gathering process. There seems to be no single correct way to collect the information needed for scanning, but at a minimum, managers must serve as the focal point.

The scanning process can be performed in a number of ways, as noted in Figure 3-2. The options shown in the figure cover a range of degrees of thoroughness and sophistication. A small organization may not have the resources or staff to attempt some of the more sophisticated approaches, whereas an institution with a large stake in successfully analyzing its competitive position should probably be doing most or all of these suggested activities. Whatever the level of sophistication, the importance of the scanning function as a source of ongoing information for strategy formulation cannot be stressed enough. Gathering information is a waste of time unless it can be used in formulating strategy. Moreover, creative ways must be devised to put information in concise and usable forms for strategic purposes.

Information for scanning should be of two types: data on the internal workings of the organization and environmental data. Data on the environment can come from many sources: reports filed publicly; federal, state, or local agency reports; the press; knowledge gleaned from managers or other personnel; trade associations and magazines; and information clearing houses, data consortia, etc. Useful information can always be obtained from published sources, but remember that in using published data, managers will often face the problem of finding that the information is too broad or too aggregated to help with institution-specific

Figure 3-2

Model of Scanning Activities

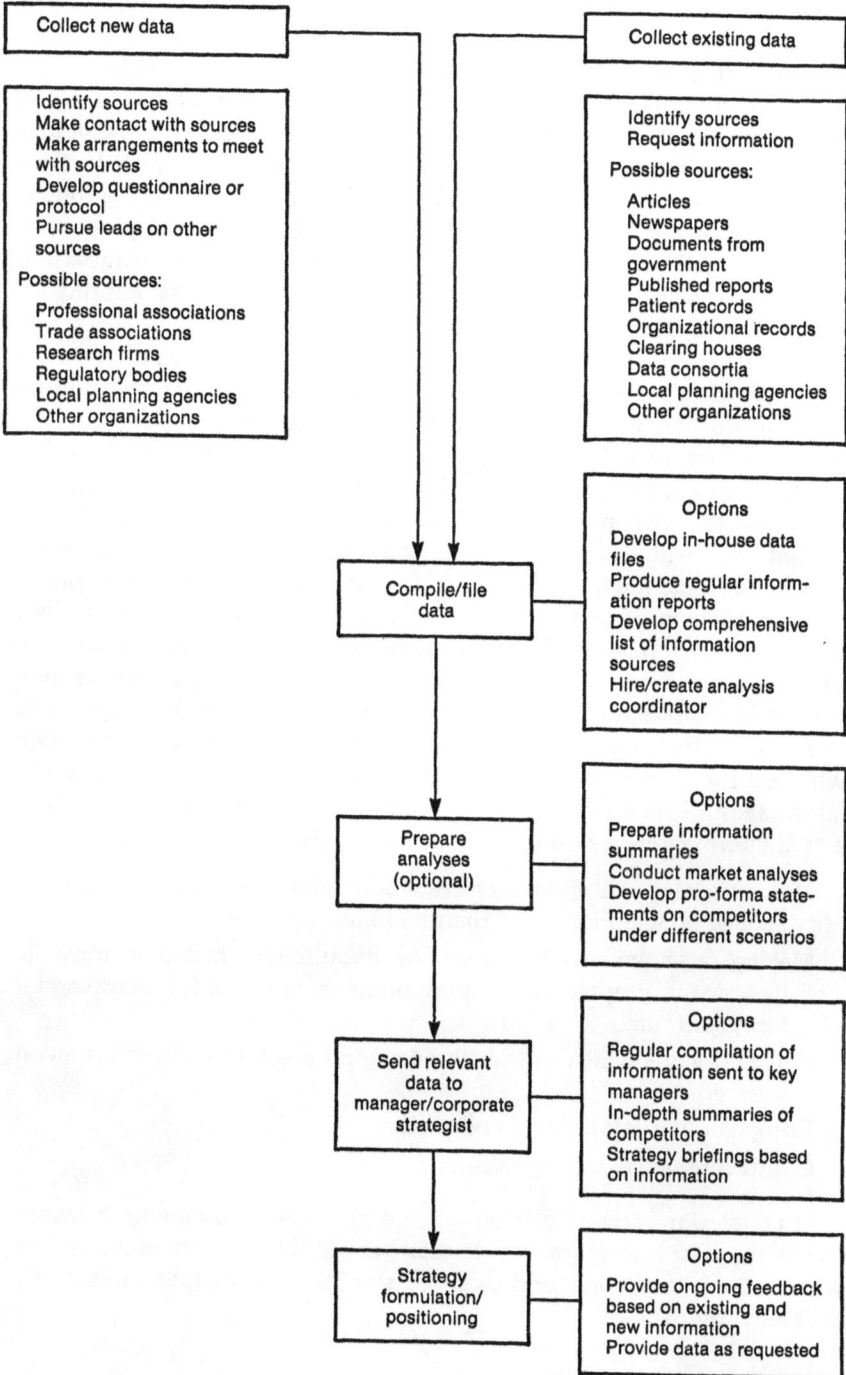

| Collect new data | | Collect existing data |

Collect new data

Identify sources
Make contact with sources
Make arrangements to meet
with sources
Develop questionnaire or
protocol
Pursue leads on other
sources

Possible sources:

Professional associations
Trade associations
Research firms
Regulatory bodies
Local planning agencies
Other organizations

Collect existing data

Identify sources
Request information

Possible sources:

Articles
Newspapers
Documents from
government
Published reports
Patient records
Organizational records
Clearing houses
Data consortia
Local planning agencies
Other organizations

Compile/file data

Options

Develop in-house data
files
Produce regular inform-
ation reports
Develop comprehensive
list of information
sources
Hire/create analysis
coordinator

Prepare analyses (optional)

Options

Prepare information
summaries
Conduct market analyses
Develop pro-forma state-
ments on competitors
under different scenarios

Send relevant data to manager/corporate strategist

Options

Regular compilation of
information sent to key
managers
In-depth summaries of
competitors
Strategy briefings based
on information

Strategy formulation/positioning

Options

Provide ongoing feedback
based on existing and
new information
Provide data as requested

analyses. Hence, published sources are better for gathering information on the general environment than for compiling data on specific competitor organizations.

Two principles can greatly facilitate access to information from published sources. First, every published source should be combed for references to other sources. Often, published documents cite individuals who are well informed, and the documents are excellent leads to other sources of information. The second principle is to keep a bibliography of everything that is uncovered. This will guard against future duplication of efforts and the agony of not being able to remember where some useful information was obtained. Summary notes on sources of information might also be developed and retained in a central file.

Managers and staff should also strongly consider the idea of gathering their own data for strategic purposes, in other words, collecting primary data. To do this, it is important to have a framework for identifying the sources of information desired, deciding what the attitude and level of cooperation are likely to be, and determining what approach should be used to obtain information. This holds true for surveys or interviews conducted both within the organization and in other organizations. Some sensitive sources are likely to be: trade association personnel who operate under a tradition of confidentiality about individual clients, and consulting firms, who may have similar constraints. Willing participants are likely to be: government regulators, planning agencies, and organizations/persons in businesses adjacent to the industry (e.g., insurance companies).

As field information is collected, attempt to speak with *key* individuals who are likely to provide useful perspectives on and interpretations of information. This also helps to cross-check and verify information. The actual information-gathering process will include:

Making contact with persons from whom information will be collected, usually by telephone and then by mail.

Making arrangements to obtain the information, including travel (if necessary), preparation of questionnaires or forms for recording information, etc.

Pursuing leads which are obtained during meetings with information sources.

Compiling the information collected.

Conducting necessary analyses.

In conclusion, scanning is one of the first major positioning activities and is the best means for you to learn about the environment and the organization, its options, and its success or failure in adapting effectively to its environment.

The risks of a narrow focus on what currently is happening, as opposed to what is likely to happen, are proportional to the rate of change in the environment which affects or potentially will affect the organization. Without the capabilities to sense environmental changes and react to them, most organizations continue allocating total energies to maintaining the status quo and, often, find themselves in serious trouble when environmental changes become so extensive that everyday operations are affected. Scanning ensures a steady and comprehensive flow of information to the adaptive subsystems of an organization, thereby allowing for appropriate organizational responses, i.e., the development of strategy.

Summary

Scanning refers to the process by which managers should gather information and analyze their organization's competitive position. Scanning is an inside-outside activity vis-à-vis positioning because, on the one hand, scanning precedes and drives other positioning activities. On the other hand, scanning is, itself, a fundamental positioning activity which must be done in conjunction with other positioning activities. Scanning provides the following:

Environmental and organizational information which identifies strategic options.

Intermediate information on organizational response to positioning activities.

Feedback to managers on the success of their strategic choices.

All organizations should scan, and should do so on a regular basis. In this era of environmental complexity and uncertainty, it is important that managers develop scanning capability in-house or else rely on consultants. To be balanced, scanning should be both internal and external to the organization. That is, managers need information on the internal operations of their organizations, as well as on the environments external to their organizations. The critical difference between the information which organizations routinely maintain and the information from scanning is a strategic focus: Scanning information is defined by the use to which it will be put.

To scan, managers (or their staff) can rely on existing and secondary information, or they can collect their own. Once information is collected, it should be maintained centrally and updated regularly. Where possible, managers should try to make forecasts of trends on the basis of scanning information to remain proactive and update strategic decisions.

Product Market Analysis

CHAPTER

4

It is always good when a man has two irons in the fire.

Beaumont and Fletcher

This chapter discusses the use of product market analysis as a positioning activity for competitive strategy. By defining market segments and the services offered, information uncertainty is reduced and resources are used in a more efficient and targeted fashion. The chapter is divided into four sections: the first section briefly reviews traditional ways in which health care managers have tended to think about and define what they offer to their markets; the second presents a systematic way of approaching product/service market analysis—"product market mapping"—which can help managers to look meaningfully at their market environments and those of competitors; in the third, marketing "quality of care" as a service attribute is addressed; and finally, the implications of a product mapping approach are discussed.

Traditional Approaches to Markets and Services

Attention to product market analysis (the term is used here to describe both products and services) is a relatively new phenomenon in the health industry. The single most significant reason for this has been the difficulty that organizations havè in defining their "health care product," or perhaps more accurately, differentiating their health products from others which, on the face of it, would appear to be homogeneous (an appendectomy is an appendectomy is an appendectomy). The difficulty in defining health products has been widely discussed in the literature, as has the critical importance to the industry of product definition, despite the problems associated with this task.[14]

Traditionally, thinking within health care organizations about product market analysis has been generated primarily by one (or a combination) of three factors: (1) the momentum of history; (2) the dictates of current reimbursement systems; and/or (3) the need to organize scarce resources. At best, however, most health care organizations have had implicit strategies about services which usually called for the organization to do or provide "more" of the same than it did last year—in terms of numbers of patient visits, patient days, or (higher) occupancy rates. Strategies emphasizing increases in services delivered were reinforced (until very recently) by the prevalence of cost-based reimbursement systems, which rewarded providers for these behaviors. Notably, because cost-based reimbursement systems provide different financial "rewards" for in-patient and ambulatory care, organizations have also tended to fragment episodes of illness into discontinuous segments of care rather than defining sets of products (services) which represent responses to stages along a continuous treatment process. Moreover, the range of strategies employed by managers was fairly narrowly circumscribed by organizational history, tradition, and perceptions of the relevant environment (Chapter 2).

An additional factor which has circumscribed thinking about product market analysis in the health industry is that historically, the role of health care organizations has been inextricably bound up with perceptions about what physicians do. As a result, thinking about what health organizations "did" has been expressed in terms of diagnostic categories treated, or severity of illness indexes for patient populations. Similarly, hospitals and ambulatory care facilities have tended to be organized by demographics (age, sex), diagnostic categories, or categories of illness severity, i.e.,

[1]M. Fottler, et al., "Guidelines to Productivity Bargaining in the Health Care Industry," *Health Care Management Review* 1, no. 4 (1979), pp. 180-85.

[2]J. B. Reiss, "Future Directions for Case-Mix Applications," *Topics in Health Care Financing,* Summer 1982, pp. 90-98.

[3]S. R. Eastaugh, "Cost of Elective Surgery and Utilization of Ancillary Services in a Teaching Hospital," *Health Services Research,* 14, no. 4 (Winter 1979), pp. 60-67.

[4]J. Yoder and R. Connor, "Diagnosis Related Groups and Management," *Topics in Health Care Financing,* Summer 1982, pp. 91-102.

acute or chronic. Recent attempts to think about "products" in more detail—as today's competitive environment requires—are generally still tied to this traditional thinking. As a result, many modern systems for health product definition or categorization depend on diagnostic categories (diagnosis-related groups) or more sophisticated attempts to measure degree of severity in patients' disorders and disabilities.

Traditional ways of defining products and services are inappropriate (and strategically ineffective) in a competitive environment. To think competitively and strategically, managers must begin to view their products in a fashion that differentiates them from products of their competitors. What does this mean in the face of seeming homogeneity, and by what means does one differentiate products beyond offering quite different ones? Managers must begin to think of their organization's services as competing in the dimensions of cost and quality and in terms of product attributes. An attribute is a characteristic, most often a distinctive mark, of a person or thing. In the marketplace, the attributes which consumers perceive different products or services to possess make a critical difference to a successful competitive strategy, for it is the perceived attributes that influence consumers to purchase one item over another. This concept is worth exploring in more detail, beginning with the general market.

A wide assortment of products varying in size, quality, reliability, appearance, and other attributes are offered in a market economy at any point in time. For some products, variety is minimal (e.g., electricity), but for most products the variety is remarkable. Consider for example, the myriad specifications for a product as simple as glass. In the service industry, which includes the health sector, variety is conceptually the most extensive, considering the need and possibility of "tailoring" services to the individual consumer. Motel guests need or prefer different sized rooms and valet and telephone services, for example. Students need different levels of educational inputs based on their interests, ability, motivation to learn, etc. In some instances, consumers face different prices for services with different attributes, while in others a common, "average" price covers all costs.

Within the industry, not all health care organizations will choose to offer the same services or, if they do, offer the same attributes to these services. Some organizations are inherently more efficient at producing one level of service than others, e.g., teaching hospitals are able to offer a different type of in-patient service than are community hospitals. By the law of comparative advantage, organizations gravitate to the attribute levels at which they produce relatively more efficiently, servicing some markets and not others. The purpose of a product market analysis is to determine which services an organization can produce at a comparative advantage over its competitors and which markets should be served.

The advantages to consumers (and producers) of providing an assortment of goods and services—in type and attributes—are obvious. Two consumers who prefer the colors red and green would both suffer from having to purchase a black Model T Ford. Accommodating their preferences for red and green Model Ts raises overall utility. Furthermore, having the ability to purchase accessories like air conditioning also increases consumer welfare, both for those willing to purchase the option and those wanting only the (cheaper) standard model. So it is with health care products and services: some consumers may prefer—and be willing to pay for—a more intensive and "luxurious" version of an appendectomy (e.g., with extensive nursing services, a private room, and color television) while others will prefer a quick, in-and-out, no-frills procedure.

A Systematic Approach to Product Market Analysis

Product attributes can only be analyzed and understood meaningfully (and competitively) in the *context of the market for which a product is intended*. An appendectomy is not simply an appendectomy, as it would be if only thought about as a product without attributes. An appendectomy done by a resident is perceived differently by consumers than is one done by a community surgeon or a teaching hospital chief, even though the outcome of the work might be identical. Similarly, the procedure is different if done in a major teaching hospital, a community hospital, or a surgicenter, even if it is done just as well and with just as much care. The costs and the added attributes (real and perceived) will also be different, and these costs and attributes become critical in a competitive situation. A businessperson, a sultan, an HMO, or a factory worker will find different combinations of cost and attributes appealing.

If you buy the same cosmetic in a luxury shop, in a department store, or at your door, is it the same? Is the experience of obtaining home health care from the Visiting Nurse Association (VNA), from a for-profit group, or from any one of a number of other associations the same, whether or not one actually gets the same care? For the purposes of competitive strategy, managers of health delivery organizations must understand how they are positioned in the market, what it is they do in the marketplace, and how the products are experienced by consumers in the markets the organization wishes to reach. The marketing mix has a mnemonic beloved of marketers—the four Ps: product, price, promotion, place. In health care delivery, there are seven Ps:

Market	Person:	What are the characteristics of the buyer?
	Problem:	What disease or problem does the buyer have?
	Preference:	What (added) attributes does the "person" desire? What does the organization offer?
Product	Professional:	Who is going to solve the problem (e.g., physician or nurse practitioner)?
	Place:	Where is the problem to be solved (e.g., hospital or home)?
	Practice:	What technology will be used (e.g., surgery or medicine)?
	Price:	What are the consequences of these factors for pricing?

This approach can assist managers in looking at market environments, reviewing products in contrast with those of competitors, and determining whether their organizations should add new products or delete/change existing ones.

The proposed approach essentially consists of four steps: (1) an analysis of who is served, and what problems they have (person and problem); (2) an analysis or map of activities produced by the organization (professional, place, practice, and price) and by the competition; (3) an analysis of the attributes of the products offered, and a matching of these with those desired by the marketplace (preference) (see third section); and (4) an analysis of the product market segment value and balance.

The first step is to analyze the market and segment it into meaningful segments, i.e., groups with distinct characteristics or problems requiring distinct approaches. Traditional marketing wisdom suggests the use of demographic, economic, or problem-type (disease) segments. Organizations like HMOs with actuarial interests, may focus on facility-use data— young, single adults differ obviously from young families or the elderly in use patterns. With a shift from the individual patient as market, to employer groups, segmenting the latter into industrial and commercial groups may make sense. (Occupational health services might be offered to the former, group rates to the latter.) Much has been written about market segmentation and is available in the literature.[5-7]

The second step involves mapping the range of products provided in a particular area by a health delivery organization or its competition. Part of this process should include definition of gaps and omissions. Mapping activities essentially makes use of three factors, two of which are shown in Figure 4-1. The first is the intensity of residential resources required in offering the product (place). Is the product to be offered in a specially

---

[5]P. D. Cooper, ed., *Health Care Marketing* (Germantown, Md.: Aspen Systems Corp., 1979).

[6]P. Kotler, *Marketing Management* (Englewood Cliffs, N.J.: Prentice-Hall, 1980).

[7]J. E. McCarthy, *Basic Marketing: A Managerial Approach*, 6th ed. (Homewood, Ill.: Richard D. Irwin, 1978).

Figure 4-1

Product Mapping

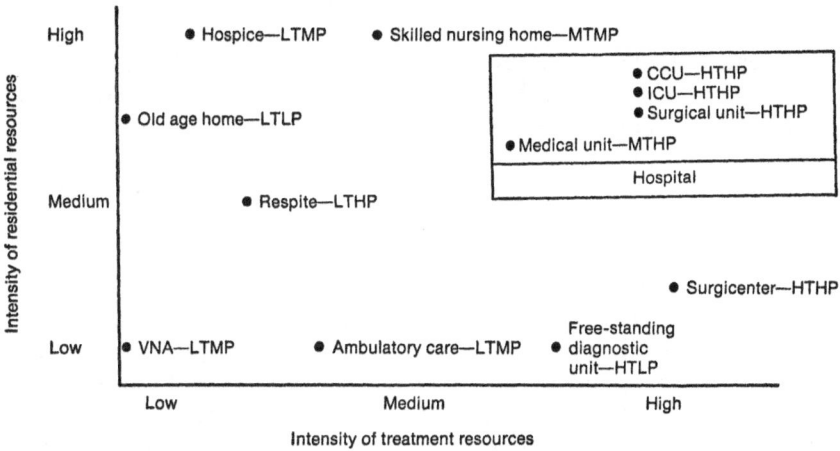

H - high.
M - medium.
L - low.
P - people; number, skill, education.
T - technology; cost and operation.

designed building, such as a hospital's intensive care unit, or at home? The critical issue is the extent to which residential resources exist (and can be intensified through further investment) or do not exist and require extensive resource outlays to develop (the vertical axis).

The second factor is the intensity of treatment resources which has, in turn, two components: (a) the intensity of technological resources (practice) required, i.e., the cost or operating expense of the technology needed; and (b) the intensity of labor resources or inputs (professional) required—number, skill level, and education. Each of these factors can be specifically costed out for a particular product (price) (the horizontal axis). A third factor (also contributing to price), is the complexity of the organizational structure required to coordinate and integrate the variety of treatment resources. Using these factors, it is possible to map out an institution's products, and/or those of the competition.

One of the critical issues in looking at environmental and competitive trends is to determine whether changes in technology make it possible to offer a particular product using a lower intensity of treatment and/or residential resources. Advances in surgical techniques now make it possible to offer diagnostic services in low-cost, low-resource settings, such as free-standing diagnostic clinics or surgicenters. On the other hand, as a result of increases in the numbers and case mix severity of the aging population, geriatric ambulatory services are becoming more complex.

Such services now require that a greater variety of treatment resources be directed towards the patient. Moreover, the intensity of services has increased, as well. The VNA, as it reviews services that previously required a relatively low intensity of residential and treatment resources, now must address a more complex and intensive mix of treatment resources. The treatment site which has been used traditionally by the VNA—the home—may no longer be the most efficient. In particular, patients' needs for occupational care, physical therapy, and supportive social services in addition to nursing care may necessitate the development of day centers or day hospitals where patients can be treated most efficiently and resources utilized most cost effectively and integrated effectively.

This type of analysis allows managers to determine whether a particular product is now being offered in the most efficient and effective manner, or whether the product could be offered more competitively in a different framework.

It should be pointed out here that a thorough analysis of the complexity and intensity of products may also require that managers measure what they do in new ways. For example, the VNA has always measured its activities in terms of patient visits—in part because reimbursement is based on number of visits but this obscures important differences between cases. As the nature of the tasks performed by the VNA has become increasingly complex new measures are needed that will differentiate different market segments. Only then can the VNA properly consider whether it should continue to serve the product market segments which it has traditionally occupied as well as those new markets that have grown up as technology has become more important. It might well be true that the major focus of the VNA's competition is a lower-technology, lower-complexity segment which, in fact, requires more marketing since it is shorter term. Should the VNA therefore compete more aggressively for these cases, or should it focus its activities more upon the higher-complexity cases, for which its particular experience may be better suited? This might then require the VNA to develop the day hospitals or day centers referred to above.

The third step is described at length in the next section. The final step assesses the value of product market segments. In an earlier chapter, a number of measures were proposed for determining competitive position and performance in product market segments. Each segment may offer a better or worse rate of return financially, and each product/service may do more or less well. But in health care, organizations may have or wish to enter market segments not for financial return but for social reasons. Every hospital takes some patients who cannot pay. A significant problem for teaching hospital group practices is that their major case load may be the indigent. And as federal supports dry up, health centers can no longer support their hitherto largely subsidized case loads. With an unfavorable market-segment financial value and poor product market financial value, such organizations must attempt to shift to other paying segments to balance their social-value segments. This can be difficult, not only because of competition but also because the types of organization and added attributes required to enter these new segments may conflict with the old segments.

Glover Clinic provides an excellent example of one approach to the problem of identifying distinctive market segments (and the need for related products). Glover Clinic is located in a state with a high birth rate. As a result, the future of obstetrics and gynecology (OB/GYN) was regarded as bright. Faced with this potential market, the new director of the OB/GYN clinic at Glover designed an innovative package of products intended to possess attributes which he felt would be competitive given the needs of the potential market. He recognized that critical issues for women were the cost of care and a more humane approach to the birth process. The director also felt that traditional obstetrical services had placed too great an emphasis on the dangers of birth and, therefore, had become too medical in their orientation. Because of the need to recognize this potential danger and yet respond to women's desires for a natural birth process, together with the desire to minimize costs, he came up with a team delivery approach in which lower-cost auxiliaries such as midwives would be used along with physicians in a collaborative practice. Given the need for a variety of roles and medical skills, the director recognized that the success of this collaboration would depend upon successfully carrying out team functions. (Recall that earlier in this discussion it was pointed out that to offer competitive products, managers may need to be willing to restructure functional areas of the organization.) The package of services that he designed included collaborative staff practice, alternative birthing centers, women's health centers, and community outreach. The alternative birthing centers were designed to be physically separate from the hospital (and thus conducive to a nonhospital environment) but still close enough to a hospital so that additional expertise was available should it be needed. Because of the emphasis on nonphysician professionals working closely with physicians, it was possible to reduce the cost of care and to have women working with women. This whole approach represents a very carefully thought out attempt to understand consumer preferences, provide related services, and create a positive image that would be attractive to women seeking alternatives to products and services offered by a traditional delivery (birthing) system. It is expected that Glover will be highly competitive with other, more traditional forms of obstetrical and gynecological practice.

Maria Nursing Home provides another example of the need to do appropriate product market analysis. Sister Fredericka has been running a nursing home providing intermediate care and skilled nursing care to the chronically and terminally ill. Her nursing home has been successful, not only because of the unfulfilled needs of this market segment and its increasing size, but also because of the special attributes associated with the care provided at the home, namely a great deal of personal and loving attention. However, Maria now needs to expand its services, since it is felt that the chronically and terminally ill offer few future, further opportunities. Moreover, the home needs to raise additional funds for an aging order of nuns requiring economic support. Where should Maria turn? Obviously, management needs to do a market analysis which identifies what needs exist among adjacent market segments. At the same time, the home should consider which of these needs Maria might supply with new services to which they can add their particular, unique attributes. Potential market segments and related products include the terminally ill (a hospice), the occasionally ill (a respite center), the well old (an old age home), or the disabled young (day center). Which of these segments they should address will depend upon the size of the segment, the extent of competition, and the degree to which they can add their particular attributes to whatever service they choose to provide.

The problem of thinking creatively about product market options also faces CEO Ken Mason as he considers the future of Midland County Hospital. He had been seriously considering collaboration and future merger. But a totally different option was presented by his vice president for operations when the latter returned from a conference at which he had heard about the activities of Henrotin Hospital and the Family Hospital of Milwaukee. Each of these hospitals was quite like Midland, a small, acute care general hospital in a highly competitive situation which it could not win. However, each hospital recognized its limitations and adopted a market-oriented approach to determining unfulfilled market needs. Henrotin started a health and fitness center which has been aggressively marketed and is expected to be not only financially viable in its own right but also a source of referral to the physicians of the hospital. The Family Hospital of Milwaukee, experiencing strong competition and without a teaching program, decided that they should not do what teaching hospitals could do better. Instead, the staff systematically reviewed a number of unfulfilled market needs and changed the focus of the hospital to one of family-oriented "total care." After obtaining trustee, staff, and community comments on possible programs (including teen pregnancy, rape, health care for the elderly, women's health, wellness clinic, medical and professional health plan, incest, domestic beatings, and sex education programs) they initially focused on two. The first was a geriatric program in which Family Hospital planned to become a regional geriatric center providing a range of in-patient, out-patient, and educational services. The second addressed the needs of the pregnant teenager. Rather than relying on physicians to provide patients, the hospital aggressively marketed its programs through newspapers, television, community groups, and school and religious organizations. The shift in social mission led to an almost immediate increase in staff, pride, and morale. Ken Mason is exploring whether an approach of this kind might be viable in his situation—recognizing that the risks were not inconsiderable, especially during the transitional period.

Finally there is the instance of the Harvard Community Health Plan. HCHP has done a thorough product market analysis and has developed, as described earlier, a differentiated (academic name, high-quality, moderate cost) brand of HMO. But as the competition from new HMOs and Independent Practice Associations (IPAs) expands and offers good, moderate-cost care, and as new blue-collar communities are entered, the differentiated image could become less effective. HCHP must decide whether to modify its successful and widely marketed brand image at all, in general, or in particular market segments.

Marketing Quality of Care

As competition in health care grows, it will increasingly take place over cost and/or quality. Generally, the issue will be cost for a given quality or quality for a given cost. Consumers want to feel that they are receiving the "best" quality care possible (absolutely or for a given price). Grasping and effectively marketing health care quality is not an easy task. What is quality of care? How is quality experienced by various concerned groups—physicians, patients, nurses, administrators, government officials? What can be done to improve the quality of care? In some form, these questions have been posed, and answers proposed, over many years. A useful definition of the quality of care is that issued by the National Institute of Medicine: "The primary goal of quality assurance should be to make health care more effective in bettering the health status and satisfaction of a population within the resources which society and individuals have chosen to spend for that care."[8]

The literature identifies a wide variety of components which form the basis for judging quality of care.[9] But despite the existence of various ways of describing and measuring quality of care, the steps to take to promote quality remain elusive in practice. A comprehensive approach on which all can agree is difficult to formulate. As a result, practical steps taken to improve care may succeed only partially, or fail entirely.

---

[8]H. R. Palmer, "Definitions and Data," in *Assuring Quality in Medical Care: On the State of the Art,* ed. R. Greene (Cambridge, Mass.: Ballinger Publishing, 1976), p. 150.

[9]R.Greene, *Assuring Quality in Medical Care: On the State of the Art* (Cambridge, Mass.: Ballinger Publishing Co., 1976), p. 3.

Another problem in defining and promoting improved quality of care occurs because what is meant by "good care" depends on who is being asked. From the patient's perspective, for example, quality of care may be good because the staff on the ward of a hospital are kind. The patient's physician may also believe that good quality care is being provided, but his or her belief is based on an entirely different measure: the low rate of infection on the ward. Both the physician and patient have reason to think that the quality of care is good, but the reasons of each are different. Despite sophisticated studies, quality of care has tended to be treated as though it were a single dimension, good or bad or somewhere in between, and as though any intervention, if it works at all, will automatically improve quality. For the reasons discussed below, this is not so.

Consider this situation: a patient does not believe he or she receives good care because the staff is shorthanded and, therefore, inattentive. The physician, too, is concerned about the patient's care: the infection rate in the ward is high. Again, each has reason to doubt the care, though the reasons are different. But what are the implications? What steps should be taken to improve quality of care? If the administration makes the decision to increase the nursing staff and encourage cheerfulness, the quality of care—in the patient's view—will improve. Yet this intervention, while valuable in one way, has in no way addressed the physican's concern; the infection rate remains unchanged.

Similarly, if stringent steps are taken and the infection rate is lowered, the physician will believe that the quality of care has improved. However, the patient, still suffering at the hands of brusque and overworked nurses, will not. Since constituents experience health care in different ways and thus evaluate care using different measures, it is not surprising that interventions to improve quality of care fail to satisfy everyone. In colloquial terms, the patient counting smiles and the physician counting incidents of staph are looking at apples and oranges.

The business literature offers a useful analog. A much replicated study found that the factors involved in producing job satisfaction and motivation are separate and distinct from the factors that lead to job dissatisfaction.[10] It therefore followed that the two feelings were *not* opposite; instead, the opposite of job satisfaction is no job satisfaction—not job dissatisfaction. The opposite of job dissatisfaction is not job satisfaction, but no job satisfaction. The study concluded that two different needs were involved: one deriving from basic biological needs and the other from the need to achieve and experience psychological growth. Dissatisfaction-avoidance factors (hygiene factors) extrinsic to the job include company policy, administration, supervision, interpersonal relationships, working

---

[10]F. Herzberg, "One More Time: How Do You Motivate Employees?" *Harvard Business Review*, January-February 1968, p. 53.

conditions, salary, status, and security. Growth or motivator factors include achievement, recognition of achievement, the work itself, responsibility, and growth or advancement.

Motivators were the primary cause of satisfaction, and hygiene factors the primary cause of unhappiness on the job. By implication, the organization must initiate different actions to address each of these two sets of factors.

These findings offer a construct with significant implications for quality of care in the field of health. The opposite of good care is *no good care* (the humane dimension) and the opposite of bad care is *no bad care* (Figure 4-2) (the technical dimension).

Figure 4-2

Four Types of Care in Health Care Units

"Bad" hospitals	Bad care and no good care	A	C
"Nice/kind" hospitals	Good care and bad care	D	A
"Good/cold" hospitals	No bad care and no good care	B	C
"Excellent" hospitals	Good care and no bad care	D	B

Bad hospitals	These demonstrate both no good care (in terms of caring) and bad care (in high infection rates, morbidity, low accreditation)
Nice/kind hospitals	These provide good care (in terms of caring) but also bad care (in high infection rates, morbidity and mortality rates)
Good/cold hospitals	These provide no bad care (adequate facilities, low morbidity and mortality rates) but also no good care (little friendliness, information sharing)
Excellent hospitals	These provide both no bad care (good accreditation, low infection, morbidity, and mortality rates) and good care (expressions of satisfaction on the part of patients, few concerns on the part of physicians).

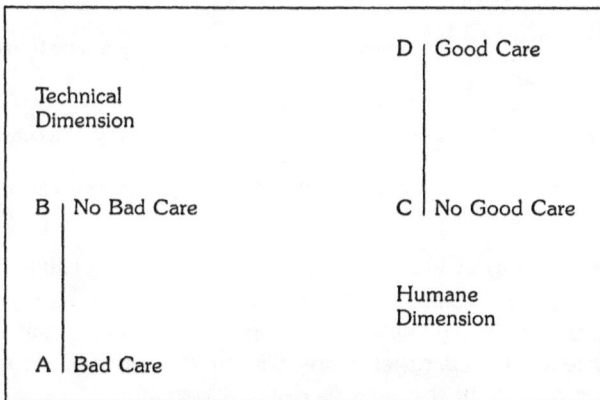

According to this construct, there are four general types of care in health units, e.g., a hospital, an out-patient clinic, a ward, etc. Assume for this example that the unit is a hospital. The characteristics of the four types are shown in Figure 4-2.

Rather few measures actually reflect good care; most reflect bad care or its absence. Changes in the factors behind these measures, therefore, are more likely to lead to an absence of bad care than to the presence of good care.

Different constituencies focus on different things: physicians, as in the early example, tend to focus on technical aspects (seeking "no bad care"), while patients want "good care," i.e., humane care. Quality—while much studied as an apparently objective phenomenon—is, in fact, essentially subjective. Good quality is more properly satisfaction with quality, bad quality is dissatisfaction.

When a hospital sets out to "improve care," that is, to make some changes that will have consequences for the patient, managers use certain mechanisms. Frequently, however, the mechanisms do not succeed—not because they fail to bring about changes, but because the changes they do bring about *fail to address the key issue behind the original dissatisfaction.*

It may be useful to present schematically a model for influencing the quality of care. It consists of four elements:

Experience of care (as an individual perceives it).

Objective measures (quantitative information on which these perceptions are based).

Factors affecting outcomes of those measures.

Mechanisms to influence the factors (and thus alter the outcomes and subsequently the experience).

To continue with one of the early examples, this is how the model works:

Physician's feelings:	"I don't feel that the quality of care here is very good."
Physician's experience:	"My last patient got infected."
Objective measure used:	The infection rate is up 4 percent.
Outcome factors invoked:	Quality of professional skills; quality of technology and facilities.
Mechanisms for change:	Increased education of staff; improved state or local regulatory practices.

The hospital, responsive to the physician's concern, initiates more advanced educational/training requirements and, in its hiring practices, builds a more technically skilled and responsible nursing staff. The state regulatory board also becomes more diligent. As a result, six months later, the infection rate in the ward is down 4 percent.

Is the care better? The doctor will say that it is less bad. The patient (to continue the original example) still complains that he or she is not getting good care because the nurses—though more technically skilled than earlier—are no friendlier.

A more useful approach for a manager's product market analysis therefore, would be one which does *not attempt to change all factors* for all people, but rather, acknowledges that there are a *variety of factors* that must be considered.

In sum, quality of care is incompletely understood; as a result, efforts to improve care often fail or succeed only partially. Quality of care continues to resist improvement because:

It is considered to be one-dimensional when, in fact, efforts to promote good care and efforts to extinguish bad care are not synonymous.

It is considered to be something objective when, in fact, it is subjective and experienced differently by different constituencies as well as by different individuals.

A single equation is used to promote change rather than the double equation that is needed.

This is summarized in Figure 4-3.

Figure 4-3

Sample of Factors in the Two Quality of Care Dimensions

	Technical Dimension	Humane Dimension
Experience (subjective)	Bad care/no bad care	Good care/no good care
Measures (quantitative)	Mortality rate Morbidity rate Infection rate Length of stay Accreditation Documentation	Compliments Complaints
Factors affecting measures/outcomes	Quality of professional skills Quality of technical facilities Quality of education	Quality and extent of information shared with patient Quality of patient/provider interaction Flexibility about rules
Mechanisms to alter factors/measures	Existence of standards Regulatory mechanisms Peer review	Development of role models Training programs Selection of staff Workload scheduling

Implications of this Approach

This approach offers managers an understanding of the different constituencies in the health care marketplace—such constituencies include administrators, physicians, other professionals, and patients—as well as of
the attributes these constituencies may regard as critical to their view of
quality of care. Professionals generally place a higher emphasis on technical quality, i.e., on the absence of bad care, while patients and some
nurses focus on the humane aspects of care. The essential issue, however, is that by understanding what these different constituencies mean by
quality of care, it is possible to: (1) design programs which will improve
quality in the direction desired by a particular constituency; and (2) market that quality of care, i.e., emphasize certain attributes so that the constituency will be pleased. Marketing quality of care therefore involves
both an objective and a subjective aspect. It is, of course, then possible to
understand what the competition is doing in relation to quality and why a
competitor's programs may be more or less successful than one's own.
Specifically, it is possible to analyze whether the competition is tapping
into or ignoring aspects of quality that are critical to constituencies.

Moreover, as competition focuses not only upon quality but upon cost,
it becomes more possible to make cost quality trade-offs (Figure 4-4). It
is generally well known that for a given investment of resources, technical
quality—whatever its particular attributes—is likely to improve only to a
certain level and then may fall off. Added resources eventually, however,
may result in unnecessary procedures and tests which simply incur costs
and do not improve or may harm the health status of the patient. It is

Figure 4-4

Relationship of Technical Quality to Investment

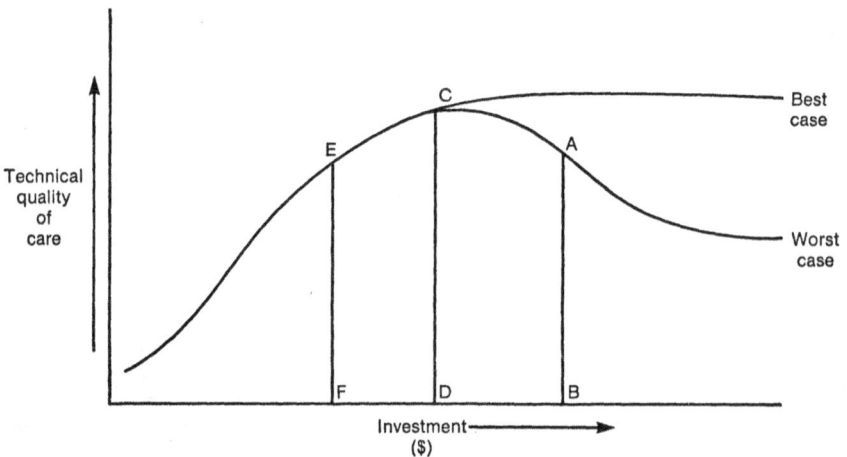

therefore possible to *reduce* the investment in quality, in terms of the iatrogenic aspects of overinvestment (from B to D). Since the curve levels out, increases in investment produce small changes in quality; therefore, it may also be possible for organizations to further reduce investments in inputs to care without incurring significant loss in perceived quality (from D to F).

Another important issue is the difference between professionals and consumers in their definition of quality. It is a problem for the VNA that its nurses are more preoccupied with the technical aspects of quality, i.e., an emphasis on no bad care, than they are on the humane aspects, i.e., the presence or absence of good care. In a competitive situation, however, if some minimal level of technical quality exists—absence of bad care—patients, consumers, and providers are likely to focus upon the "good" i.e., humane rather than "bad" aspects of performance. Thus, providers will probably be much more concerned about their patient being seen promptly and regularly than about whether a bandage is being tied properly or a leg has been moved 15 instead of 20 times for rehabilitative therapy. Similarly, patients will be concerned about being seen regularly and with some personal concern. If the VNA is to compete effectively, its nurses' efforts must be redirected toward attributes and behaviors which the provider and the patient regard as quality. The VNA must then consider its own concerns with quality and make the appropriate trade-offs.

This approach to product analysis also affords a clear way of competing in terms of the best quality for a given price, or the best price for a given quality. This is not possible if managers fail to see the importance of determining what quality means. By doing market research and discovering exactly what attributes are associated with quality in a constituent's minds, programs can be clearly and specifically oriented towards satisfying these concerns.

Designing a Market Research and Action Program: The Focused Target Program

The purpose of focused target programs is to identify the factors which various constituencies identify as crucial components of the quality of care. Then, working with the two-dimensional construct, and using research findings that more finely discriminate among the factors that affect quality of care, several focused target programs (FTPs) can be designed.

Gathering Information on the Constructs of Care   Begin with the hypothesis of the two-dimensional construct (Figure 4-3). You will want to document individuals' own assessments of care without leading them, and thus you will ask five kinds of questions. To ensure that people

Specific Program Objectives of an FTP

To identify and document those factors which various constituencies in health specify as crucial to quality of care.

To attempt to identify new and useful measures of good care.

To develop recommendations based on the project results that will be useful to health delivery organizations in planning interventions to improve care, and in marketing their products.

are reflecting on the same or very similar experiences, ask about care on a particular unit over the past three months. Ask questions such as:

What is your experience with care in this unit?

What do you feel constitutes good care? Bad care?

How do you judge it? What evidence do you have?

What measures do you use in considering that evidence?

What organizational efforts make a difference to care?

Ask these questions of individuals in six major groups (these groups represent constituencies):

1. Physicians.
2. Nurses.
3. Patients.
4. Senior staff (nonmedical).
5. Government officials.
6. Families.

To be most effective, try to interview 6 to 10 people in each of these groups. As a result of these interviews, three levels of information will be made available:

Factors that each group believes affect the quality of care. (It will be useful to check these factors against the two-dimensional matrix.)

Evidence on which each group bases its opinions.

Relationship of opinion to objective measures.

Formulation of Questionnaires   On the basis of the preliminary information gathered in these interviews, you or your staff can formulate questionnaires. Each questionnaire should contain a core group of questions asked of individuals in all six groups; in addition, there may be some questions that are specifically tailored to one or another of the groups. For example, it is possible that similar questions may be framed in technical (rather than lay) language for physicians, and lay (rather than technical) language for patients. The difference is in linguistic style rather than in substance. Another difference may be in the complexity of questions asked. Questions about measures of quality may use simple constructs for one audience and more complex constructs for another to elicit more detailed information. At this time, too, you will see whether some of the questions lend themselves to quantifiable measures to facilitate data analysis later on.

Testing the Instruments   These questions can be tested with both original and new interviewees, to find out whether the questions seem useful in discerning aspects of care and whether the questions can be easily answered.

Clarifying the Sample   Once the questionnaire is developed, also ascertain the possibility of obtaining aggregate responses: Do all individuals in a group of nurses or patients, for example, give the same or very similar answers? The answers may vary widely among individuals in a constituent group; that will mean that the pilot test must include a large number of people in each group to obtain an accurate assessment of care in a particular organizational unit, such as a ward or out-patient unit. If, however, the answers are fairly uniform within a group, a smaller number of people can be questioned to obtain accurate information. There may be clusters of similar responses among the categories; it is unlikely, however, that they will overlap a great deal. Presumably, the constituent groups, as suggested earlier, are responding to different attributes.

The purpose of this approach is not to force an overall rating of the ward or out-patient unit based on some average of points, but rather, to develop a *profile* of the organizational unit and use it as a diagnostic tool in assessing the need for change and the factors to be addressed.

Design and Implementation of an FTP   In setting targets for change based on the questionnaires, specify whether the change is expected to promote an increased experience of "good care" or to lessen the experience of "bad care." Specify, too, which group or groups are expected to experience the change. Therefore, in setting targets for change consider the following:

Degree of departure from current behaviors/operations.

Relative importance of the opinion of the group which will experience the change.

Amenability to change of various organizational factors.

The cost of developing and implementing alternative organizational mechanisms.

Clearly, trade-offs are always involved in effors to improve care, and a detailed cost-benefit analysis is essential. Hospital administration (one particular constituency) may need to accept improvement that falls short of the degree desired because, at the margin, the "final 10 percent" may be too expensive for the improvement it produces. A needed improvement may also be postponed indefinitely because it involves factors that are highly resistant to change. Factors within the jurisdiction of a particular ward, for example, may be more easily changed than general factors which can only be changed by intervention from the higher administration of the hospital. Taking these theoretical and pragmatic factors into account, you can develop organizational mechanisms that will result in change in some selected factors.

Summary

With the growth of competition and of resource and information uncertainty, it becomes imperative for health care providers to be able to deliver what the consumer wants at a price the consumer can afford. More educated consumers are more critical and more demanding. And the buyer is no longer simply the patient or the referring physican, but often another health care delivery organization. This chapter addresses the issue of product market analysis, pointing out that products can only be analyzed in the context of a marketplace which contains the demand for certain kinds of care and certain kinds of attributes. A way of mapping health care products to ascertain the competitive marketplace is elucidated; this includes the dimensions of intensity of residential resources, technical resources, skill inputs, and the need for organizational integration. A two-dimensional approach to marketing the quality of care is set forth, emphasizing that improvements in one dimension will not result in improvements in the other. The use of focused target programs as a way of economically addresing market segment needs is described.

Collaboration: Match or Miss

We all come down to dinner,
but each has a room to himself.
Walter Bagehot

The subject of this chapter is collaboration between two or more institutions, which may result in what is referred to as a multi-institutional system. It is remarkable how even major institutions entertain collaboration, which may determine their future, and yet fail to address key issues. The result of failing to deal with key issues may be the breakup of a potentially fruitful endeavor or costly prolongation of the process. The Brigham and Womens Hospital of Boston merger took 12 years to bring off. In that time, the cost of the new buildings the three hospitals wanted rose from $40 million to over $100 million. In other instances, institutions with nothing in common waste time and money only to discover that collaboration is neither desirable nor feasible.

The chapter is organized into the following parts: first, the utility of collaboration as a response to environmental uncertainty is discussed; then the chapter presents a three-phase approach by which managers can assess whether or not to enter collaborative arrangements with other institutions and what the potential problems are in the transition toward collaboration. A model of the developmental stages of collaboration follows in the third section. Included in the model is a discussion of the issues and problems that managers may encounter as they attempt collaboration. Finally structural alternatives are presented.

Why Collaborate?

Collaboration can be considered as one type of response to the problems of uncertainty and complexity discussed in Chapter 1. As legislators show a greater propensity to regulate health care costs, as consumers' expectations become more sophisticated, as community representatives demand a part in the planning process, and as available funds become more limited, collaboration increasingly makes good sense. At a minimum, it allows health care organizations to determine a greater amount of their own fate, by initiating and working with other institutions rather than being controlled by external factors and regulations. In a now feverishly competitive health environment, hospitals and other health care delivery institutions can seek advantages by combining their resources and/or markets through collaborative ventures. Essentially this is the intent of collaboration: to gain a competitive edge; to seek to dominate an existing market; to enlarge a market; or to gain access to a new market(s).

For some institutions, collaboration may be altogether critical to survival. This is not to say that most health care organizations now favor collaboration over autonomy. It has not traditionally been in the interest of individual institutions to work together, and the goal of protecting one's self-interest has not diminished or changed; self-interests must simply be attained differently in the new environment. For many institutions, collaboration may be the only reasonable action given the environmental and financial pressures, though competition may continue, even with collaborating partner(s) alongside.[1]

Unfortunately, too many managers of health care organizations explore collaboration less on the basis of a particular objective identified as part of a well-defined strategy than because they are seduced by the idea or philosophy of collaboration. Collaborative ventures which are not oriented to meet clear-cut objectives or which do not recognize that competition/collaboration must coexist tend to be time-consuming and costly. They take a very long period of time to bring off and may be less than totally successful. Some fail altogether. In fact, it is extremely difficult even to judge the "success" of collaborative arrangements, because the collaboration can be cost-effective in the sense of saving money for member organizations and yet be considered "unsuccessful" by staff members who feel alienated within the new arrangement. A good rule of thumb is that if a collaborative arrangement continues to exist for five years or

---

[1]D. Barrett, *Multihospital Systems: The Process of Development* (Cambridge, Mass.: Oelgeschlager, Gunn and Hain, 1980).

more, it has been successful.[2] Clearly though, the fact that an "effective" collaboration may be hard to actually document means that managers must enter them with prospective strategic goals in mind to avoid trying to justify (retrospectively) having entered the collaboration by pointing out that it has been "a success."

Making Collaboration Work

What are the critical factors that determine success or failure in collaborative ventures and how can the likelihood of success or failure be assessed by managers? Three sets of factors are important (Figure 5-1):

Figure 5-1

Factors Which Affect the Success or Failure of Collaboration

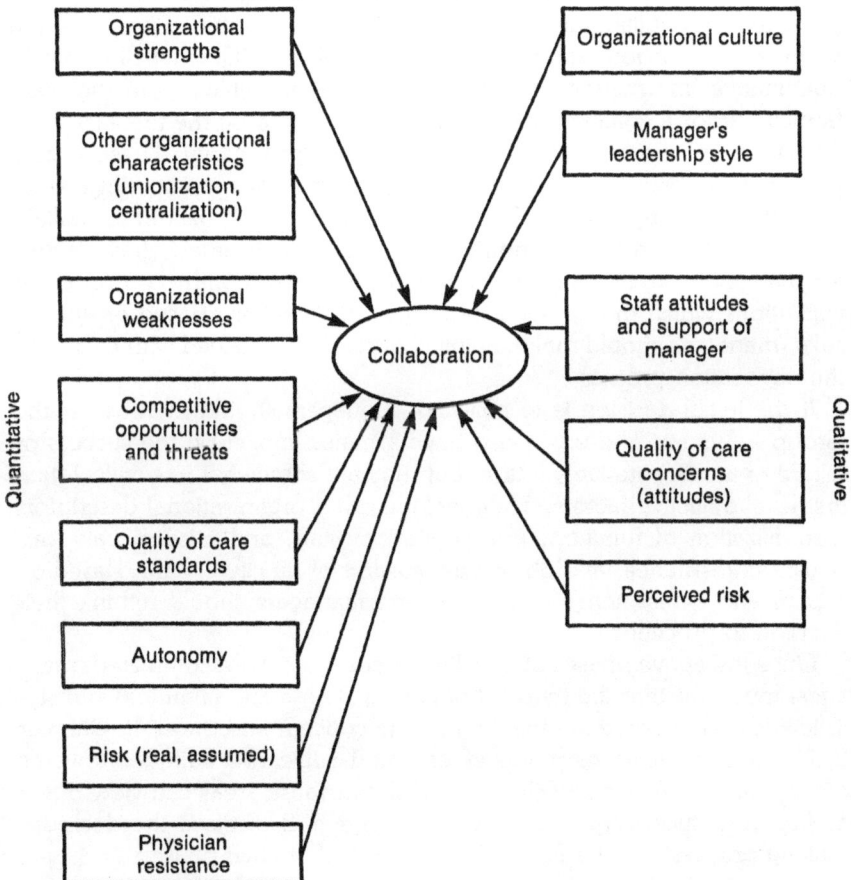

---

[2]Barrett, *Multihospital Systems*, p. 28.

Group 1 Identification of a rationale for collaboration—assessment of competitive needs, existing resources, and new, feasible activities that might be of mutual interest.

Group 2 Identification of forces for/against collaboration in each institution that might affect the likelihood of successful collaboration.

Group 3 Identification of style complementarity or conflicts that might smooth/hinder the collaborative process and may need to be either resolved or factored into any proposed structure.

External pressures notwithstanding, the success of a collaboration will usually depend on the "goodness of fit" or complementarity between two or more organizations. To assess the degree of complementarity, a three-phased decision-making process for managers is proposed, the results of which will give a strong indication of the desirability of proceeding with plans to enter collaboration with another organization(s). Phase I of the process involves both an internal and external scan (Chapter 3) to obtain quantitative information on the Group 1 factors which form the basic framework for a collaboration and are also likely to be the first factors to "break" a collaboration if there is poor complementarity. These factors include organizational needs, organizational strengths, competitive situation, type and degree of risk that each organization will bear in the collaboration, and need for autonomy. Managers should assess these factors for their own organization and compare the results with data on other institutions which may participate in the collaboration. Based on the results, managers should make an initial decision to proceed with or call off the negotiation process.

If the initial decision is to proceed, managers should then assess the Group 2 factors. These will also have a major impact on the success or failure of a collaborative venture, but they are somewhat less critical than first-level objective factors. They include other organizational descriptors (centralization of function, unionization of staff, and mission balance), physician resistance, and objective measures of quality of care. Based on a scan and assessment of these factors, managers should rethink their decision to proceed.

Once the above phases of deciding to collaborate are completed, managers must consider the third set of factors. These are attitudinal and stylistic and include organizational culture (a concept introduced in Chapter 2), leadership, style of management, and subjective attitudes towards quality of care. Incompatibility in any one of these areas can slow down or hinder a successful collaboration. Figure 5-2 displays the decision-making process and the factors to be assessed at each phase.

Figure 5-2

Deciding to Enter Collaboration

Phase I   Group 1 Factors
              Complementarity of needs
              Complementarity of strengths
              Competitive situation
              Autonomy
              Risk

Make initial decision to proceed based on the above

Phase II   Group 2 Factors
              Centralization of functions
              Unionization of staff
              Mission balance
              Physician resistance
              Quality of care (objective measures)

Make decision to proceed based on the above

Phase III   Group 3 Factors
              Organizational culture
              Leadership style
              Quality of care (subjective attitude)

Rationale for Collaboration (Group 1 Factors)

Group 1 factors are indicators of the complementarity which exists among various objective characteristics of those institutions contemplating a collaborative arrangement. These factors tend to be quantifiable and can be assessed using objective measures and (usually) available data. For example, if the objective of collaboration for one institution is to increase its access to a certain market segment, it then would be inappropriate and ineffective for that institution to collaborate with another institution which is also lacking access to the desired market. This factor can be readily determined by looking at institutional service data.

An essential part of planning for collaboration must involve: (1) identification of needs; (2) identification of strengths; and (3) ensuring that the identification of (1) and (2) is grounded in objective measures rather than subjective impressions. The scanning process, which was described in Chapter 3, should provide information on the strengths and weaknesses of other institutions in the relevant environment (external scanning), as well as objective data on the strengths and weaknesses of the institution contemplating collaboration (internal scanning). Using these objective data, managers can develop a "collaborative profile" to see what collaboration with another organization might look like in *practice* as opposed to theory.

A close study may reveal that what initially appeared to be a promising venture is not so promising after all because, in fact, the institutions turn out to have the same strengths or weaknesses. Where the latter is true, a collaboration is doubling the vulnerability rather than the competitive muscle of each. (Occasionally, of course, institutions proceed anyway. Political considerations may supercede the practical considerations of the market place; but even then, lack of complementary profiles cannot be ignored because they will continue to be an issue.)

The first order of business for institutions contemplating a collaboration must be to take a hard look at what they can do, what they offer, and what they need. The enticement of a collaboration is always that two (or more) partners should be stronger together than they could hope to be separately; therefore, each must believe that a collaboration would enhance its existing profile by adding new strengths without diminishing existing ones. (Or at least, not diminishing them very much; compromise may well turn out to be the order of the day.) Certainly, though, no collaboration can prove successful if one of the partners is convinced that it has lost more than it has gained. Developing a profile of complementary health and management services offered, of markets served, is the ideal.

Clearly, the precise advantages and disadvantages of collaboration for each institution need to be identified and assessed using objective data. If, for instance, improved management services is the key point, a lack of improved clinical services may not matter at all. Actual deterioration may be an offsetting factor, but if there is no deterioration in services—and no improvement—then the focus on management strengths can be maintained.

In identifying strengths and needs, it is important to distinguish between those objectively measured and those subjectively felt. The board of an institution may feel that expanded services would be a good idea, and yet an analytical study of the market may indicate that there is no market for expanded services. In such a case, a perceived need turns out to be just that—a general longing, unsupported by existing evidence.

Collaboration works better, overall, when institutions are reasonably equal—none has marked weaknesses (comparatively speaking) in capital, operating revenue and costs, or capacity to borrow.

Given that the purpose behind all collaborations is an increase in competitive edge, it is important for institutions in the exploratory stage to map out the marketplace (through scanning) and clearly specify what they hope to gain (strategic objectives). An institution may already be feeling the press of competition and be looking to acquire additional resources to meet the competition. Hill Medical Center (HMC), a sizable hospital, expects to offer a greater range of services to smaller hospitals and an improved quality of management through its collaboration with Dale Medical Center (DMC), another hospital in an adjacent, but not competitive, region.

In the case where managers view collaboration proactively, the real pressures of competition may still be down the road. DMC, looking to the future, wants to be able to compete with the resources of any for-profit group which might come into its area. HMC currently has "dogs snapping at its heels," in the form of local competition. So, although the time frame is different, each institution feels the need to shore up against encroaching competition.

At the same time, the fact that two or more institutions join together is no guarantee that the competition will be overcome, even if the match is close to ideal. Indeed, collaboration may actually bring about the very situation institutions are trying to avoid; it may precipitate a merger of other smaller, competing institutions to create an even stronger competitive entity. When this occurs, the initial collaborators may be no better off than they were originally. The chain reaction is obvious; any new collaboration appears stronger to its competition—and it most likely is stronger. In the eyes of its competitors, it becomes a force to be reckoned with and they will reckon with it, possibly through a collaboration of their own. Thus, in assessing competion, it is necessary for managers not only to accurately measure the competition that exists but also to keep a weather eye out for competition that may emerge in response to the managers' actions.

Amid all the pressures for collaboration that exist—and despite common interests, needs, and a competitive edge—collaborative arrangements may still falter because of organizational resistance to loss of autonomy. Autonomy is best measured in terms of fiscal decision making, and it is usually this power that institutions are least willing to renounce. Scenarios are frequently observed in which two institutions appear ready to collaborate—even merge—in every other way and yet remain reluctant to combine their assets.

Some institutions choose to combine forces to carry out certain projects and still remain fiscally separate. This solution creates a confounding problem, however. One of the distinct advantages of merger or other strong forms of collaboration is that the combined sum of assets of two or more institutions gives the new organization a far stronger borrowing capability than any of the parts could have alone. If a stronger line of credit or an improved bond rating to finance new efforts is a major motivation behind the merger, forfeiting that advantage may leave the new partners with many of the difficulties of collaboration and none of the big rewards.

In other cases, institutions may feel that they are being forced to forego their autonomy—that is, their fiscal control—before they have found out whether they can work well together in harness. It is at this point that the need clearly arises for some established "courting" procedures wherein potential partners can try out a joint venture to see how well they do. The French proverb that admonishes, "Do not attempt a marriage together until you have attempted to cook an omelet in one kitchen," becomes surprisingly apt. The omelet experiment, for health care institutions in the trial stage of collaboration, may be specific and involve joint ventures such as shared services. Another venture might be financial: putting some—but not all—assets together into a holding company, not an operating company.

It is the rare collaboration that offers no downside risk. There are the easily noticed and quantifiable risks of losing control over an important matter—often fiscal—central to running the institution, or of one partner truly giving up more than it is getting (as opposed to simply feeling that way). There are also shadow risks that do not arise until talks of collaboration are fully under way; for instance, in the DMC case, the possibility is that the merger might precipitate the kind of giant opposition, in the form of a competing collaboration, that the center was trying to avoid. A more common risk (see below) is that of the flight of fearful physicians to some competitive institution.

Risk assessments for each institution call for a thorough review of contingencies, an honest statement of what risks are unacceptable to management, and what loss of control is too much for an individual organization to accept. One hospital, for example, may care so strongly about quality control that any partnership which appears to threaten its ability to maintain its high standards would be seen as unacceptable. For another institution, the risk of extending financial liabilities in the form of debts or runaway operating costs is unacceptable. For a third, it may be the fear that the new corporation would take over a particular function, such as centralized financial reporting and data processing. Or, because of incurred risk and anticipated loss of power, an institution may find that it is simply unable to relinquish control. If institutions can identify significant compatibility in their areas of strengths, needs, potential risks, and competitive situation, Phase I of the decision process is completed and an initial hurdle has been passed. Figure 5-3 is a checklist of the types of questions which managers should answer in Phase I, comparing their answers with those of other institutions to offer a preliminary compatibility profile. The first "judgment call" about whether to pursue collaborative arrangements between two institutions should be made only after these questions have been answered.

Figure 5 - 3

Checklist of Phase I Questions for Collaboration

Markets
> To what extent do markets served by each institution overlap or complement each other?

Products and services
> To what extent do the services of each institution overlap or complement each other?

Identified needs
> What is the objective assessment of needs not now being filled for each institution? (Subjective needs assessments can be developed, but they are less meaningful at this stage than are quantifiable needs.)

Identified strengths
> What are those particular areas of distinctive competence in each institution? In which areas do they have management slack? What can they provide to other institutions?

Financial situation
> What is the financial situation of each institution in terms of capital and operating revenues and costs? In particular, what financial problems does each have and what capacity to borrow?

Competitive situation
> What is the competitive situation of each collaborating institution and what is its objective in exploring collaboration? Will collaboration improve or exacerbate the situation?

Willingness to commit assets/autonomy
> Since one potential advantage of collaboration involves the commitment of assets and improved capacity to leverage debts through obtaining an improved bond rating, what is the willingness of each institution to relinquish autonomy to gain this advantage?

Risks
> What real risks will be assumed by each institution as the the result of collaboration? Does one institution have significantly more to lose (or gain) than another? What critical functions for each institution are vulnerable ones for which collaboration may mean some unacceptable risk or loss of control?

Identified potential economies of scale
> Potential collaborating institutions may have invested in certain functions which would become more cost effective or revenue producing if combined on a larger scale with those of other institutions.

If the collaborative profile passes this initial hurdle, the next level of objective (quantifiable) factors should be considered.

Forces for/against Collaboration (Group 2 Factors)

Other organizational characteristics to assess include potential centralization, the mission of the organization, unionization, physician resistance, and the quality of care.

Centralization refers to the extent to which any potential activity lends itself to being provided in a consolidated way. On the one hand, centralization can reduce duplication of effort and gain economies of scale. On the other hand, decentralizing ("unbundling") some services, especially selected clinical services, enables an institution to reach more (and diversified) market segments (Chapter 6). Some functions lend themselves to centralization, e.g., computer services, communications programs, certain specialized medical services. Other functions do not. Even for services which lend themselves to centralization, there are other factors which will determine, in the final analysis, whether centralization is desirable and/or feasible. For example, for institutions in close geographic proximity to one another, specialized clinical facilities can be widely shared through a centralized source. Transportation distances, however can pose major problems that prevent centralized services for institutions which are physically far apart (e.g., DMC and HMC).

If distance is one concrete factor, philosophy is another factor, more amorphous but equally compelling. Some institutions—such as teaching hospitals—pride themselves on research, and they allocate staff and financial resources to research and training. For others, such as community hospitals, the mission is oriented to primary care services, and the hospitals spend their dollars to raise the quality of these services. Institutions which focus on one mission frequently have a difficult time accommodating the goals of institutions which focus on another. The "mission balance" between potential partners, as much as miles or known needs and strengths, is a factor that can promote or dissolve a collaboration.

The question of mission leads to the question of physicians, and the potential resistance of the physicians in each institution to collaboration. The hospital affiliated with a medical school is likely to have attracted and retained a body of physicians that is different—in skills, interests, and focus—from those in a community hospital primarily concerned with high-quality primary care. The mode of practice favored by these different groups of physicians also plays a part; those in single practice may well be more wary of collaboration than those who participate in a group practice and, therefore, use many of the principles of collaboration. The extent to which physicians know about collaborative possibilities, and favor (or do not favor) them matter. Where there is a low level of physician knowledge, or unfavorable attitudes (either based on little knowledge or knowledge of other collaborations which have gone awry) the physicians may feel threatened and actively oppose what the administration of the institution hopes to achieve. Physician resistance can be a real barrier. If it exists in an institution considering collaboration, the leading proponents would do well to attend to the resistance and carry on awareness sessions designed to offset it rather than to ignore it.

The degree of resistance often varies according to the existing quality of the physician/administration relationship. Do physicians feel they have been included adequately in past strategic decisions? At DMC, for instance, physicians tend to feel that in the past, they have not always been consulted about issues which directly concern them.

Physician resistance also varies with the nature of the collaboration. In the case of HMC, this resistance may not turn out to be a significant factor, since the partnership would focus on management activities rather than on patient care. (Clearly, the latter is the purview of physicians, and where patient care is concerned, physicians can be expected to react strongly.) This is not to imply however, that physicians may not develop strong feelings about nonclinical issues. If physicians feel their needs and those of their patients are being ignored in a new concern for bigger laundries, the physicians may prove to be a formidable barrier after all.

Major questions for proponents of collaboration are when and how much to involve the physicians in the process. A small, outspoken group of physicians opposing collaboration does not necessarily represent the whole group. In fact, physician reaction may vary quite widely within an institution. The majority may be somewhat uninformed and can often be swayed either way.

Physicians are not the only constituency in the health care setting capable of weighing a decision toward or away from collaboration. Another key point is whether the institutions are unionized. If one is and one is not, unionization can become a major stumbling block. However, the state of unionization and employee attitudes toward it, is often more significant than the fact of unionization alone. If one institution is not unionized and its employees are opposed to unionization, they may create serious obstacles to collaboration with an institution which is unionized. On the other hand, if employees of one hospital are not presently unionized but do not feel strongly one way or the other, plans for a partnership may push them, willingly enough, to unionize.

The final issue in this second set of factors is the question of quality of care. Some aspects of this always important issue relate to style, and these are discussed below. But other aspects do not. For example, is an institution affiliated with a medical school? If it is, then the quality of care question has an academic stamp, and for such an institution to collaborate—even short of merger—with a nonaffiliated institution may be seen as a distinct lowering of institutional standards. DMC wanted to set up its own nursing school, but DMC's physicians detected in this proposal a potential lowering of standards set by a medical-school-affiliated nursing school.

Quality of care carries legal implications, as well. In a collaborative effort, the institution with the highest existing quality of care is the one that may establish the legal standard. For example, three teaching hospitals (with very high standards) and eight community hospitals (whose standards were not as rigid) were proposing to join together to create a cancer care network. Some of the physicians in the community hospitals had concerns that if the plan went through, they would be forbidden to carry out certain procedures in certain ways in their own hospitals.

Figure 5-4 presents a checklist for managers to use in addressing the Group 2 factors that affect collaboration outcomes. As in Phase I, managers should complete Phase II by reassessing the potential success of the collaborative relationship.

Figure 5-4

Checklist of Phase II Questions for Collaboration

Capacity to centralize
> What functions lend themselves to centralization to gain economies of scale? Is centralization possible? (e.g., are large geographic distances involved?)

Mission balance
> What is the emphasis of each institution in the areas of research, teaching, and service? Institutions focusing on one of these may have difficulty in collaborating with other institutions focusing upon another.

Physician resistance
> To what extent do doctors in each institution have information about collaborative prospects? Are attitudes favorable or unfavorable towards collaboration? What roles do physicians play in governance of each institution?

Unionization
> To what extent is each potential collaborating institution unionized or not?

Quality of care issues
> What is the emphasis in each institution on technical or human quality factors, and in particular to what extent is quality of care identified with academic affiliation? (e.g., institutions affiliated with medical schools may feel that their quality of care would suffer in collaboration with institutions not so affiliated.)

If the first phase or exploration of collaboration suggests that there is a nice mesh between what one institution offers and what another needs, and the second indicates that collaboration is still a viable possibility, a third question arises: In spite of the needs each seeks to fill and the strengths each brings, and even if the forces are favorable, will the attempted collaboration ultimately flounder because the operating styles of the two are radically different?

Complementarity of Style (Group 3 Factors)

The third set of factors that determines the success or failure of collaboration are qualitative and provide signals on how well the styles of two (or more) institutions will match. "Style" addresses a number of factors.

All organizations have their own distinctive histories and, over time, an organizational culture evolves which reflects this history: the staff that work in the organization; the groups it embodies and the vested interests they have created; and the way in which the organization has adapted to its environment in the past.[3] Collaboration necessitates changes in that organizational culture which may or may not be well received by the organization's membership. A key task facing managers during collaboration is to infuse the process with value to mobilize staff energies and direct them towards the objectives of the collaborative arrangement.

For example, functional centralization within each institution, different from geographic centralization (discussed earlier), is an important style factor. To what extent does each institution value control, loyalty, and autonomy, and how will that mesh conflict with the values of another partner? And what are the attitudes toward quality of care? Two institutions with equally strong reputations for care may encounter differences of opinion on clinical procedures because one views quality of care as primarily a technical matter and the other emphasizes its humane aspects.

The profile of attending physician attitudes, too, is important. Within the organization's culture, are physicians oriented academically or clinically? What kinds of rewards do the physicians in each hospital expect: salary, fee for service, other incentives such as profit sharing? And how involved in the decision making of top management do physicians feel? Are there mechanisms in place for managing the manager-physician relationship, or do the two groups tend to meet rarely and then, most often, over a dispute? These factors may have an impact on physician resistance, discussed under Phase II factors above; however, they are grouped with stylistic descriptors because they strongly reflect the intraorganizational roles and the "world view" of staff, both of which may be significantly different in different institutions.

Not only do organizations have certain cultures or "styles," but so do their managers. Style is an amalgam of the assumptions that a manager makes. Managers make assumptions about the staff they employ, the mission of their organizations, etc., and these assumptions affect a manager's performance and form the basis of his or her leadership style. A manager's leadership style, in turn, leads him or her to decisions about how the organization will relate to its larger environment, including other organizations. If leadership and/or organizational styles do not match well, collaboration may be impossible. How an institution sees itself may be crucial as more factual considerations (e.g., is one hospital focused on research

---

[3]See for example, A Decade of Implementation: The Multiple Hospital Management Concept Revisited, National Forum in Hospital and Health Affairs (Durham, N.C.: Duke University, 1975); M. Brown and B. MacCool, eds., Multihospital Systems: Strategies for Organization and Management (Rockville, Maryland: Aspen Systems, 1980).

while the other is not?). The question of style—in terms of both leadership and organizational culture—cannot be underestimated. Finally, what is the corporate culture of the management group itself? There may be powerful and prevailing myths about the CEO and the top managers that percolate throughout the institution and create certain expectations: Is this an institution that meets change head on and aggressively, or is this an organization that only changes when it must and then at a snail's pace? *Perceived* management style—aggressive and ready to grow, or passive and reactive—will also affect staff attitudes towards collaboration.

The way in which information is shared, decisions are made, and tasks and responsibilities are asigned all color institutional style. An institution with leaders who are aggressive and ready to change, who allocate decision-making authority to the staff (ultimately responsible for decisions), and who clearly define tasks and responsibilities, may have difficulty entering a relationship with an institution in which the CEO is conservative, decisions are made in a top-down fashion, and information sharing is considered an unnecessary luxury. Conservative leaders will find conflicts in style with leaders who feel that decisions should be made in a diffusely democratic fashion and all information shared with everyone, whether they need it or not. Similarly, the institution that rewards its managers on the basis of performance may encounter great resistance to new ventures on the part of a management that rewards on the basis of seniority. A checklist for collaboration, then, must include style consideration (Figure 5-5).

Projecting the Transition

Managers should be aware that once collaboration is entered, a transitional period will occur which is likely to be stressful for the organization. This period will be marked by different problems for each institution. Managers should anticipate, and be prepared to address, four major issues:

1. Staff Effects of Uncertainty Period and Risk In the stage during which merger is being considered, managers, staff, and physicians may all deal with uncertainty in various ways, including considering and making alternative moves. The risk of a prolonged uncertainty period must be assessed and steps taken to minimize such risk. To what extent is management developing mechanisms to ease "transitional trauma"? If hospital physicians shift patients to a competing hospital, the bargaining position of the hospital may be significantly altered. If good managers leave unnecessarily, the collaboration will be that much more difficult.

2. Collaboration Workload Collaboration generally involves an addition of workload, especially for senior managers. To what extent is

Figure 5-5

Checklist of Phase III Questions for Collaboration

Background of managers
> To what extent are top management "home grown" or "imported"?

Performance expectations and measurement
> To what extent are managers clearly rewarded for performance as opposed to seniority or other factors?

Quality of care attitudes
> To what extent in each institution is there an emphasis on the technical or human aspects of quality of care?

Risk attitude
> With regard to critical decision making about finances or medical matters, what are the attitudes of the chief executive officer, the top physicians, and the board with regard to the taking of risks?

Physician orientation
> To what extent are the physicans academically or clinically oriented?

Physician remuneration
> To what extent are physicians in each institution paid by salary or fee for service, and to what extent do other incentives exist?

Physician autonomy
> To what extent is the prevailing pattern of practice in each institution individually oriented, group oriented, or institutionally oriented?

Physician/administrator relationships and mechanisms
> What is the quality of the physician-administrator relationship in the institution, and what are the major methods of handling it? Do these in fact exist or are they absent? Do they involve discussion or involvement of the physicians in critical decisions through critical roles?

Task clarity and responsibility
> To what extent are the tasks of management clearly defined and responsibility allocated to individuals as opposed to vague definition and lack of clarity regarding responsibility?

Delegation regarding information and decisions
> To what extent is information shared among management in an institution and are decisions delegated?

Decision style
> How much is the prevailing way of making decisions among management group oriented and participative or individually oriented?

CEO orientation
> Is the chief executive officer an academic, an administrator, or a physician?

Centralization
> Is management style centralized or decentralized? (To what extent does a manager truly delegate/share operational responsibilities?)

Management depth
> With regard to skills, experience, training, and general or parochial attitudes, how thin or deep is the management of an institution?

Management myths
> To what extent are there powerful and prevailing myths about chief executive officer and the top managers that may influence attitudes?

Management style
> To what extent is the management style aggressive and growth oriented as opposed to passive or reactive?

such addition recognized and rewarded (positive), or expected without remuneration (negative)?

3. Capacity to Develop Transitional Organizational Policies and Procedures   Generally, the step between an autonomous institution and a collaborative venture requires the setting up of various forms of transitional mechanisms to make decisions about and manage the collaborative process. To what extent are institutions ready and capable of delegating responsibility, time, and money in the creation of such necessary management processes?

4. Agreement About Top Jobs   Is there clear-cut agreement about who will do and have what in the new venture? This simple question, if negative, brings progress to a grinding halt. When two hospitals formed a holding company, for instance, each CEO wished to run the new enterprise. The eventual (interim) solution was a joint presidency: the CEOs make policy together, but each has a complementary and distinct operating role. Arriving at this solution took six months' work and the problem was really postponed.

Collaboration: How to Go About It

Once managers decide that they should collaborate, the question becomes how to do so. The model presented below, derived from case studies and other work over the years, suggests four developmental stages of collaboration.[4] Issues of concern for managers at each stage of development are included in the model. These issues represent tasks that must be addressed if the collaboration is to proceed smoothly and successfully. The reader should note that this model includes only those activities which are necessary to implement collaborative arrangements; it assumes that managers have completed the three-phase decision-making process described above, using the suggested checklists, and have determined that it would be desirable to enter into a collaborative arrangement.

Stage 1: Forming the Multi-Institutional System

The earliest questions that those wishing to set up a multi-institutional system need to resolve are:

---

[4]A. Sheldon, *Managing Change and Collaboration in the Health System* (Cambridge, Mass.: Oelgeschlager, Gunn and Hain, 1979).

Which specific organizations should be invited to join?

What should the statement of purpose be?

In fact, those questions are interactive and need to be answered simultaneously. This is shown schematically in Figure 5-6.

Figure 5-6

Forming a Multi-Institutional System—Stage 1

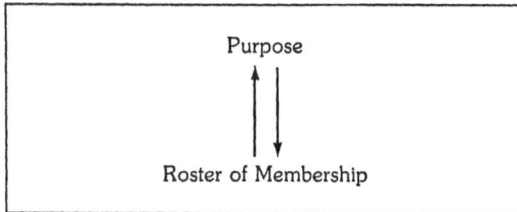

Given a particular formulation of purpose, one can logically deduce the list of organizations that should be a part of the collaboration. By contrast, it is conceivable that independent factors may bring a particular set of institutions together. In such an event, the purpose would evolve from consensus among the institutional representatives. But there should be a purpose which can be fulfilled by action. Stage 3 work, designing activities, may require redefinition of purpose, and thence of membership, since the original actors may no longer be relevant.

Situation-specific characteristics thus seem to play a major role in how the purpose and the roster of membership evolve. What does not seem to be situation specific, however, is a normative statement of the long-term direction in which this evolution should proceed.

A long-term vision of purpose and membership, however, can at best be only a guide to more short-term decisions. Situation-specific factors will have a significant bearing on these decisions. The most relevant criterion for short-term decisions on purpose and membership seems to be: Strengthen the facilitators and weaken the barriers to the development of collaborative relationships—at least until the collaboration builds up a critical momentum of its own. One major step toward meeting this criterion is the development of norms among the institutional representatives whereby these individuals regard each other and their institutions as strong, competent, and equal. (This was discussed in the previous section, but merits repetition here. Managers should be able to use quantitative/objective information to determine and document strengths and competencies for other member organizations.) Viewed from this perspective, the leadership should avoid creating a situation in which one particular instituiton is viewed as a burden on other institutions. In other words, institutions that are weak—in either competence or finances—should not be invited in; or if they are, then the stronger institutions must be willing to help the weaker institutions become strong.

Stage 2: Developing the Decision-Making Mechanisms

Once a multi-institutional system has been formed, either formally or informally, the basic issue is: which individuals will relate to each other and how (Figure 5-7)? More specifically:

Figure 5-7

Forming a Multi-Institutional System—Stage 2

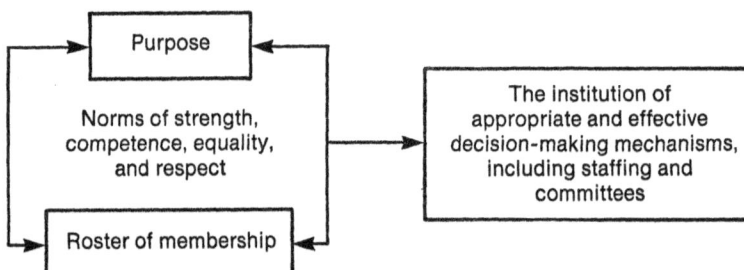

Which individuals from the member institutions should be invited to participate in the collaborative decision-making process?

What forms/committees should be created in which these individuals can meet on an ongoing basis?

In the event of conflicts of loyalty/opinion on the part of two or more of the institutional representatives, how should these conflicts be resolved and decisions made?

This phase is crucial, since the potential loss of old identity, with no new one yet emerging, means a heightened need for some anchors. Anchors may well take the form of a transitional structure and/or process that is to be trusted as the new shape forms. No trust, no progress. Staffing design may be critical.

It hardly needs mentioning that the three policymaking elements of most health care organizations are: trustees, administrators, and physicians. All three groups have considerable strategic power within each organization. It is therefore necessary that individuals from these three constituencies in every member institution interact with their counterparts from the others. Whether decision-making forums mix these, or keep them distinct, is to some degree a matter of taste or habit.

Accordingly, in many successful health collaborations, the board consists of a trustee, an administrator, and the chief of medical staff (or similar physician representative) from each institution. Furthermore, three standing committees of board members of the consortium exist—one of trustees, one of administrators, and one of the medical chiefs. The administrative and medical committees may further set up task forces to examine key issues individually.

Finally, competitive roles must be dealt with. People who represent institutions in a multi-institutional organization play dual roles or have multiple constituencies as responsible members of their own institution and as executives in the multi-institutional organization. At times, decisions may be required that place them in a potential conflict situation. Unless they have dealt with these dual roles, have thought about the consequences of this problem in terms of action, and have established relationships of trust and power with their own constituencies at home, the multi-institutional organization will begin to crumble.

Stage 3: Taking Concrete Action

A multi-institutional system exists to get things done. Accordingly, the basic issues at Stage 3 are:

What mix of activities should the collaboration take up for concrete collaborative action?

In what order should these activities be taken up?

Are activities new and nonthreatening, or do they raise questions about a total realignment of the member institutions? Do they enhance competition in undesirable areas?

From all the possible activities, the leadership must help members select a subset in which priorities reflect the overall purposes of the multi-institutional system. These activities must be backed up by commitment from the participants, who must act according to these priorities. This commitment may take the form of backing up difficult actions, of committing resources, or of committing time. It may also include securing stability for the collaboration by obtaining long-term funding. The appropriateness of the mechanisms of decision making developed in Stage 2 will be reflected in the quality of the action taken in Stage 3.

The process of sorting out priorities for action may well begin with a decision to use a *programmatic approach* for the generation and discussion of substantive issues. Under this approach, a particular program such as rehabilitation/cardiac care/cancer care is taken up for scrutiny in its entirety. This helps focus attention on the improvement of all aspects of health care delivery within that particular program. Benefits are many:

It helps bring out gaps in the existing system.

It helps specific institutions and the multi-institutional organization in providing rational arguments in support of certificate of need (CON) applications to fill these gaps.

By appealing to consumer-benefit values, it makes it more likely that member institutions will agree to close down/relocate some of their existing services.

It provides a rational framework for involving health providers serving the same geographic area but not officially within the multi-institutional organization.

If a decision to use the programmatic approach has been made, the next step is to decide on which programs to take up. This decision should be based on a judgment of the historical barriers and facilitators to the development of collaborative processes existing within the consortium and its environment. The "program" chosen should provide valuable experience to the consortium in using the programmatic approach; on the other hand, it should not be too explosive, otherwise, the consortium may fall apart before any concrete learning has taken place. The revised sequence of activities now looks as shown in Figure 5-8.

Espousing the need for a successful health collaboration and creating one through concrete action are two very different phenomena. In the short run, some institutional leaders may have to "bite the bullet," i.e., forego short-run benefits for their institutions in return for greater long-term autonomy from regulatory agencies. The tendency may be to avoid doing so by picking up trivial "programs" for concrete action during the initial phases, or picking up new activities that do not raise questions of realignment. While this makes a collaborative setting less threatening to member institutions, it also breeds frustration and makes it increasingly difficult to tackle the more conflict-ridden programs. After having begun with relatively trivial programs, most collaborations have undergone a period of crisis in which the participants feel very frustrated with the achievements of the organization. Progress will occur only if the hurt of not going ahead (threat of bankruptcy, loss of sevice, etc.) is more than the discomfort of proceeding. All members must hurt for matters to proceed, i.e., the old must be discounted for the new to be adopted. In many collaborations there is failure to progress at this point because:

No sanctions evolve for actions on the part of individual institutions that would encourage cooperation with the goals of the group.

Figure 5 - 8

Forming a Multi-Institutional System—Stage 3

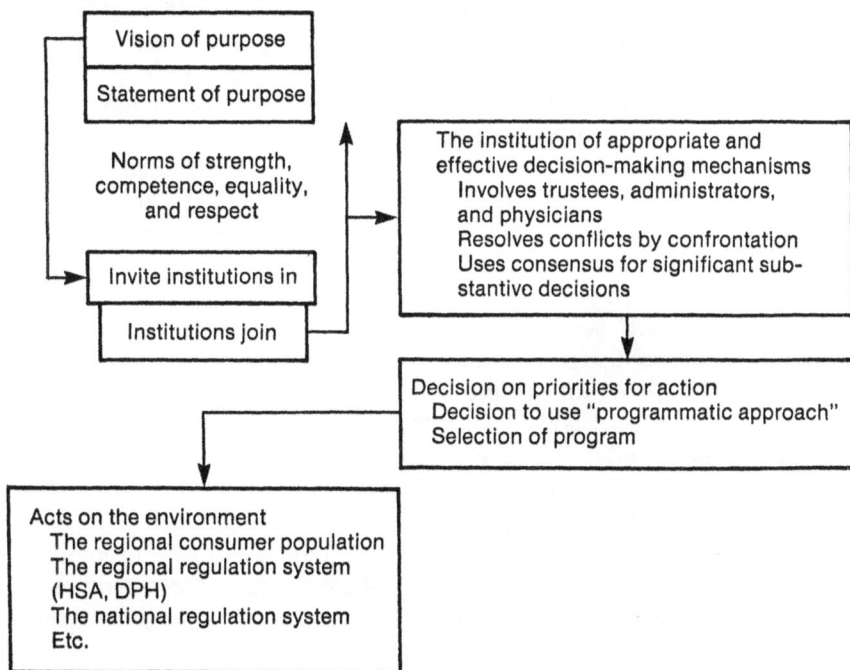

```
┌──────────────────────────┐
│    Vision of purpose      │
├──────────────────────────┤
│   Statement of purpose    │       ┌────────────────────────────────────────┐
├──────────────────────────┤       │  The institution of appropriate and     │
│    Norms of strength,     │       │  effective decision-making mechanisms    │
│   competence, equality,   │       │     Involves trustees, administrators,   │
│      and respect          │       │     and physicians                       │
├──────────────────────────┤       │     Resolves conflicts by confrontation  │
│   Invite institutions in  │       │     Uses consensus for significant sub-  │
├──────────────────────────┤       │     stantive decisions                   │
│    Institutions join      │       └────────────────────────────────────────┘
└──────────────────────────┘
                                    ┌────────────────────────────────────────┐
                                    │  Decision on priorities for action       │
                                    │     Decision to use "programmatic approach" │
                                    │     Selection of program                  │
                                    └────────────────────────────────────────┘
┌──────────────────────────────────┐
│  Acts on the environment          │
│     The regional consumer population │
│     The regional regulation system  │
│     (HSA, DPH)                    │
│     The national regulation system  │
│     Etc.                          │
└──────────────────────────────────┘
```

The low level of commitment on the part of membership leads to little or no confronting behavior; thus, issues remain superficial and non-controversial.

Each institution is anxious to maintain the status quo and acts to ensure that its own interests will not be subsumed by the interests of the whole.

It is at this stage that it may be necessary to revisit Stages 1 and 2 and revise membership, purpose, and decision mechanisms as the definition of purpose becomes clearer through the definition of action.

Stage 4: Consolidation and Integration

Stage 4 involves moving beyond collaboration to some structural and process alteration that involves reallocating resources more efficiently toward redefined goals.

One approach to integration and consolidation that is effective is the use of staff task forces to recommend areas for possible improvement. Since it is the middle staff level that best knows what the problems are and has the relevant information, these may be brought together, by function, to recommend potentially fruitful collaborative activity and consolidation. Often this level, while threatened, is enormously creative in proposing activities not likely to be considered by top management. Brigham and Women's departments recommended merger when top management was thinking in terms of joint venture. The Health Corporation of the Archdiocese of Newark completed some 18 departmental reviews across its three hospitals with potential savings running into the hundreds of thousands of dollars.

Integration and consolidation comprise a commitment to a new paradigm, and they will generally only work for those collaborations of the closer kind. Where there is reallocation of resources, there must be some form of integration, and in the environmental conditions earlier described, this is most likely to take the form of the creation of a multiorganizational matrix. There will likely be centralization of some functions.There is also likely to be a redefinition of the market in light of the enhanced capability of the aggregated and redeployed resources. Thus, for example, Baptist Hospital in Memphis, Tennessee, having joined a group of equally large hospitals, now considers its market to extend as far south as New Orleans, 400 miles away, a considerable enlargement over the previous market.

Why will integration probably take the form of a matrix? The matrix is the preferred structural choice when three basic conditions exist simultaneously:[5]

1. Pressures for Shared Resources

Where organizations are under considerable pressure to achieve economies of scale and high performance utilizing scarce human resources and meeting high quality standards, there is a clear indication to adopt a matrix.

2. Pressures for High Information-Processing Capacity

If the demands placed on the organization are changing and relatively unpredictable, large amounts of new information must therefore be assimilated and responded to in a coherent way. Such uncertainty in the external environment calls for an enriched information-processing capacity within the organization. The more interdependence there is among people, as in condition 1, the greater the information-processing load. Uncertainty, complexity, and interdependence all generate a need for infor-

---

[5]S. Davis, and P. Lawrence, *Matrix* (Reading, Mass.: Addison-Wesley, 1977).

mation-processing capacity, which is enhanced by the matrix form of organization. This is not simply a matter of increasing the flow of reports, briefings, and informal communications through the information system, but of weighting the significance of the new information and making decisions that commit the organization to a successfully adaptive response. More people must be in a position to think and act as general managers, and this is the kind of behavior that can result only from the matrix form of structure.

3. Pressures for Dual Focus   Finally, where organizations have outside pressures to maintain a dual focus, the matrix is the preferred form. In health as in aerospace, there is a need to focus both on the customer or patient and on complex, technical issues.

The evolutionary sequence of a successful collaboration is expected to proceed as shown in Figure 5-9 with one caveat: often Stage 4 is never reached.

Types of Multi-Institutional Collaboration

There are many forms of collaboration—many structural types, each with its corporate character and legal peculiarity.[6] This section breifly delineates the major types (Figure 5-10) and then summarizes the advantages and disadvantages of selected collaborative arrangements.

It should be stated that in reality pure types rarely exist. Most organizations are also rarely involved in a purely collaborative relationship with another institution. Usually they are mixed relationships, with both collaborative and competitive aspects. An understanding of the various forms which collaboration can take clarifies the strategic advantages of one approach over another and should also provide the reader with useful background information for subsequent discussions of the success of collaborative ventures and the developmental stages of collaboration.

Federation

A federation is formed when several institutions incorporate for such purposes as exchanging information, sharing services, and eliminating duplication. This is a very limited approach toward collaboration, and is very informal. Cooperation is totally voluntary. Institutions involved tend to be located within the same city or general area and to draw their pa-

---

[6]Sheldon, *Managing Change.*

Figure 5 - 9

Developmental Stages of Collaboration

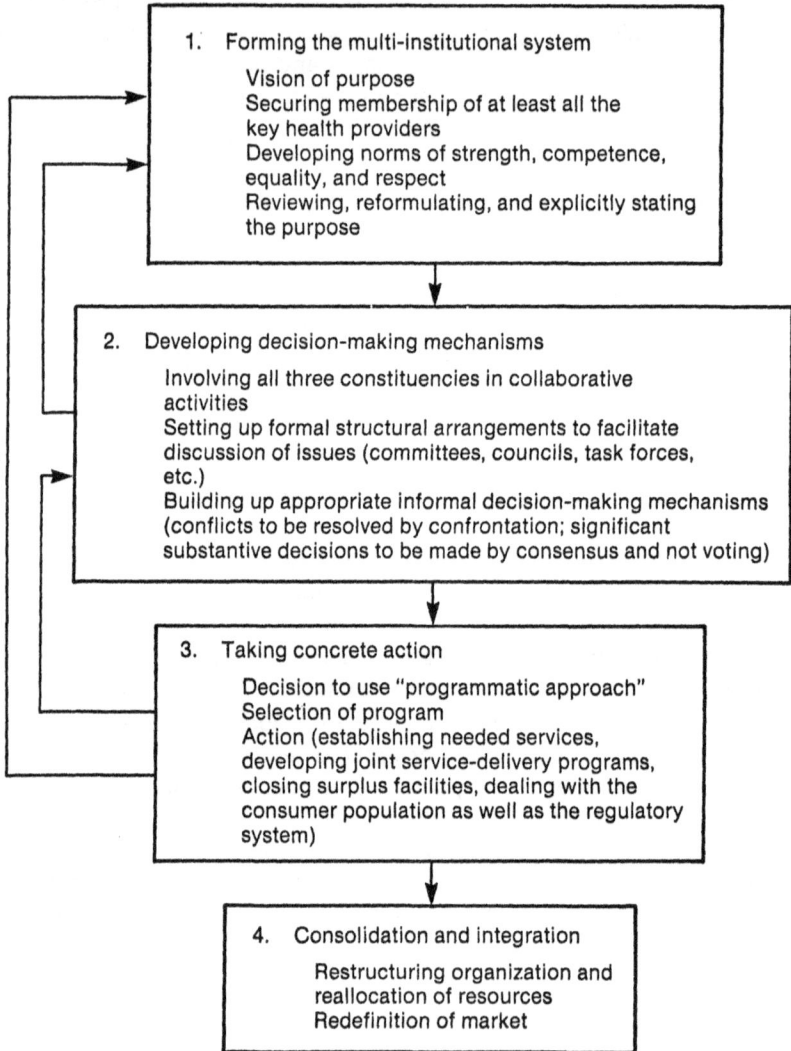

```
┌──────────────────────────────────────────────────┐
│  1.  Forming the multi-institutional system        │
│                                                    │
│        Vision of purpose                           │
│        Securing membership of at least all the     │
│        key health providers                        │
│        Developing norms of strength, competence,   │
│        equality, and respect                       │
│        Reviewing, reformulating, and explicitly    │
│        stating the purpose                         │
└──────────────────────────────────────────────────┘
```

```
┌──────────────────────────────────────────────────┐
│  2.  Developing decision-making mechanisms          │
│                                                    │
│        Involving all three constituencies in        │
│        collaborative activities                     │
│        Setting up formal structural arrangements    │
│        to facilitate discussion of issues           │
│        (committees, councils, task forces, etc.)    │
│        Building up appropriate informal decision-    │
│        making mechanisms (conflicts to be resolved  │
│        by confrontation; significant substantive    │
│        decisions to be made by consensus and not    │
│        voting)                                      │
└──────────────────────────────────────────────────┘
```

```
┌──────────────────────────────────────────────────┐
│  3.  Taking concrete action                         │
│                                                    │
│        Decision to use "programmatic approach"      │
│        Selection of program                         │
│        Action (establishing needed services,        │
│        developing joint service-delivery programs,  │
│        closing surplus facilities, dealing with the │
│        consumer population as well as the           │
│        regulatory system)                           │
└──────────────────────────────────────────────────┘
```

```
┌──────────────────────────────────────────────────┐
│  4.  Consolidation and integration                  │
│                                                    │
│        Restructuring organization and               │
│        reallocation of resources                    │
│        Redefinition of market                       │
└──────────────────────────────────────────────────┘
```

Figure 5-10

Types of Collaborative Arrangements

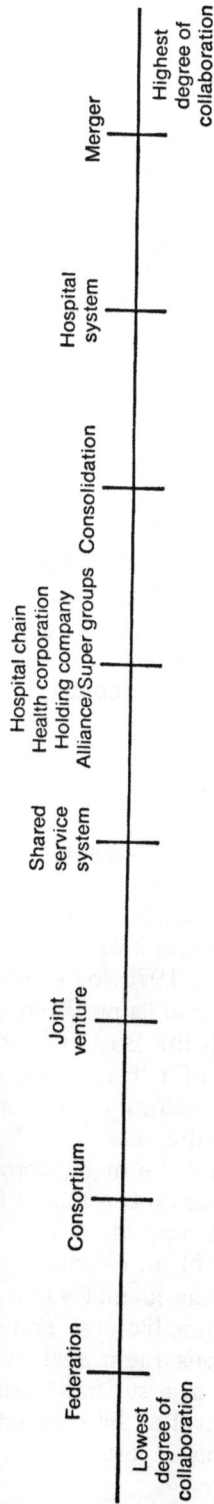

Federation · Consortium · Joint venture · Shared service system · Hospital chain / Health corporation / Holding company / Alliance/Super groups · Consolidation · Hospital system · Merger

Lowest degree of collaboration — Highest degree of collaboration tients from the same population. They may compete with one another or share some services. The institutions are distinct, with separate identities and physical facilities. Each institution retains its separate medical and administrative staffs and maintains separate budgets. Each has its own board of directors.

A federation usually sets up a board that includes the administrator, one trustee from each institution, and one public member. Meetings of the board may be irregular and are seen as a way of getting the administrators and trustees from each participating organization to know one another better and to increase understanding of the others. There is no special federation staff. A federation does not provide for any special planning mechanisms, such as a committee, other than the board. External pressures, particularly government regulations, seem to be the major impetus for this type of collaboration.

A federation has no clout. Consequently, there are very few achievements other than the provision of a forum for informal discussions. By allowing representatives from each institution to get to know each other better, it can set the stage for developing a higher degree of collaboration. The fact that federations commit little and do less has made them less popular than other forms of collaboration.

Consortium

Examples of consortia are the South Middlesex Hospital Association (SMHA) in Cambridge and Somerville, Massachusetts and the Capital Area Health Consortium (CAHC) in Hartford, Connecticut. The former comprises five acute care hospitals and two chronic/rehabilitation facilities. SMHA was formed in 1975 to "promote collaborative solutions to common problem areas," and its proximity to Boston has led association hospitals to compete with the Boston hospitals. CAHC was created in 1974 through the signing of a "Hartford Compact." The consortium was created to collectively maintain, improve, and develop a health care system to meet the needs of the area.

While consortia are still not a highly committed form of collaboration, this arrangement is more advanced than a federation because the members often pay dues that support, in part, a salaried consortium staff. Usually this staff consists of an executive director and some assistants. The members have separate identities and physical facilities. All are located within a given geographic area and draw their patients from the same population. The consortium staff may be housed in one of the member organizations or in a separate facility. The location of the staff can be crucial to the survival of the consortium.

Each member retains its separate board, medical and administrative staffs, and budget. The executive board of the consortium usually consists of trustee, medical, and administrative representation, and it may meet monthly. There are often special committees to the board, including a planning committee. Institutions usually form a consortium as a response to increasing government regulation (external factors), they feel that be standing together they can increase their power against outside intervention and become some kind of lobby. The major (and often only) advantage of a consortium is that it allows its members to get to know one another better. Like a federation, it can promote nonthreatening programs among its members and provide those members with shared services, depending on relative strength and commitment. A consortium board has no clout other than peer pressure. The fact that it has a staff and its members pay dues puts it at a more advanced stage than a federation, although the two may, in fact, be quite similar. And for similar reasons, a consortium is becoming an infrequent form of institutional collaboration. It promises collaboration across the board—unrealistic in most instances.

Joint Venture

The joint venture corporation is formed for a specific rather than a general purpose and therefore limits collaboration to this purpose. The members have separate physical facilities and each member has two identities, one apart from and another together with other members. Each has its own board, administrator, medical staffs, and budget.

There is a separate board that consists of medical, administrative, and trustee representatives, and the staff may be housed in one of the member facilities. The presidents of each of the member corporations and the CEO of the joint venture corporation are in the top management positions. Committees to the board involve member representatives. While the members share the specified services and can therefore reduce duplication, they retain their individual identities. This is a useful device for focusing on mutual interests while keeping competitive issues apart.

Shared-Service System/Management Contracting

A shared-service system provides services for and/or manages all or parts of a group of health care facilities. The members retain their separate identities and separate physical facilities. The participants are independent and serve distinct communities. Each retains its separate board, medical staff, and budget.

The reason for establishing this type of arrangement may be a need on the part of individual institutions to improve management structures; but more often, the reason is to facilitate purchasing services at reduced cost and sell the services to outside markets. Clinical services are not usually involved at all. This arrangement is very popular. Again, it acknowledges mutuality of interests, but as a separate corporation, keeps competitive issues at a distance.

Hospital Chain

A chain is owned and/or operated by a single corporation in which centralized services are provided to the individual hospitals. Chains tend to be more common in rural regions, since they provide a way for small hospitals to obtain economies of scale. Usually, participating hospitals are independent, and each hospital both retains its separate identity and takes on the corporate identity. Individual medical staffs are also maintained. An administrator who reports to one of the corporate officers is assigned to each hospital, and each hospital retains a separate board. Decisions are made at both the corporate and local levels, and planning is done at both levels, also.

Health Corporation

A group of hospitals may also join together to form a health corporation which is similar to a chain. Usually they do so in response to internal pressures, such as financial difficulties, rather than to external pressures. The hospitals tend to be independent from one another and are usually located in distinct communities. Corporate officers are housed in a separate facility. Each participating hospital retains its separate identity and at the same time takes on the corporate identity. Each hospital has its own medical staff, and all decisions regarding patient care are made locally. The corporation controls the hospitals' budgets and holds "reserved powers," which give it ultimate authority over budget approval and program and service development. Each hospital is responsible for its own planning. Many religious orders with dispersed hospitals have turned to this arrangement to obtain the advantages of centralized management or, for example, to improve their bond ratings. For-profits also favor health corporations.

Holding Company

A holding company owns a group of institutions and controls their fiscal affairs, while it leaves the actual operations and day-to-day decision-making responsibilities to the individual institutions. Each organization retains its separate facility and identity, while also assuming the corporate identity. Individual budgets must be approved by the holding company. Assets and operational budgets are held jointly. A public relations department and a planning committee may be maintained at the corporate level. This is increasingly popular as the form, par excellence, which creates collaborative flexibility without completely diminishing individual autonomy. It may be set up to hold the assets of the members or to institute another new set of activities.

Alliance/Super Groups

Super groups and alliances are usually created by several multi-institutional groups; they take the form of a "macro" holding company or joint venture, or less frequently, one of the other corporate forms described above.

Consolidation

When health care institutions consolidate, their administrations merge (totally integrate), while the clinical services of each institution may still remain intact. This system works best when the institutions are of different types and there is no overlap of clinical services—for example, adult and children's facilities. Each facility retains its separate identity and also assumes a corporate identity. The medical staffs remain separate. Each member retains its own board, which becomes a division of the corporate board. The budgets for each member are set at the corporate level. Major decisions are made by a single, central administration. There is usually a planning committee that reports to the corporate board. Consolidation may be difficult to achieve even in a tightly held corporation, because of the resistance of historically distinct hospital entities.

Hospital System

In a hospital system separate institutions become divisions of a larger system. This arrangement can be brought about when one hospital purchases another and/or constructs another, the facilities remain physically distinct, but their separate identities are lost, are subsumed by that of the larger system. There is usually one medical staff, with all of the physicians having an obligation to rotate through all the divisions. There is also one administration that can be housed in any one of the member facilities. The divisions serve a distinct patient population and offer a similar range of services. The hospitals share and refer patients among themselves. The assets of the divisions are held centrally, while the operating budgets are controlled at both the local and system levels. Ultimate decisions regarding finances, planning, and development are the responsibility of the corporate board. A separate planning committee usually reports to the board. Unlike the situation with consolidation, there is also usually a single board rather than separate divisional boards. A system is similar to consolidation in that it maintains no separate corporate staff (as in a hospital chain or holding company), but has only the regular corporate structure of a single institution. This is commonly found, for example, among Roman Catholic hospitals.

Merger

A merger represents the highest degree of collaboration. It is the total integration of two or more institutions into (usually) a new institution with a new identity, although acquisition (absorption of one organization by another) is included in this category.

In this form of collaboration, individual identities are totally surrendered. Separate physical facilities and medical and administrative staffs are eliminated and replaced by one facility, one medical staff, and one administration. Since this type of collaboration usually results in the elimination of jobs, it is difficult to accomplish. Mergers can also be difficult to achieve because the separate institutions may resist having to relinquish their identities. This type of arrangement is likely to be most viable when the organizations involved are in extreme financial difficulties and are faced with the choice of either merging or closing.

Advantages and Disadvantages of Forms of Collaboration

The single most critical issue in discovering the optimal form of collaboration, given any situation, is to determine the degree of competition between collaborators on the one hand, and the activities intended, on the other. Only then can a structure be created that recognizes the one and facilitates the other. Collaboration is a means of improving an individual entity's competitive position. (Already formed voluntary hospital groups may aggregate further into so-called supergroups—often corporations of amazing size, e.g., 37,000 beds and $1.5 billion annually in revenues.) It is therefore a delicate matter when several institutions seek association, since what they do together must help each in their unique situation, if the association is to endure.

The looser forms of collaboration suffer from a dual problem. They tend to emphasize collaboration across the board but are not sufficiently stable or committed to be very effective at doing anything concrete. Joint ventures are very useful for specific concrete action, requiring that members commit support to the project. Usually these are single projects. Shared-service systems are fine if the content of what is to be done is known ahead of time. Holding companies give a great deal of flexibility, as they may hold the assets of members or simply be a vehicle for undefined future projects. Management contracting or shared-service systems are useful and concrete ways of starting collaborative ventures that may broaden later to more intimate forms of association. Often a management contract leads to subsequent acquisition. Chains, corporations, and holding companies are often the characteristic forms for broad, multihospital collaborative systems, where central managerial capability is important but clinical autonomy is untouched. Commitment of assets facilitates access to the capital market at favorable rates. Mergers and consolidations are more intimate forms, where both managerial and clinical integration are intended. More often than not, one form precedes another, and no single form will necessarily be the best one for every stage of any association.

It must be stressed that competitive analysis, as outlined in Chapter 2, is a necessary precursor for each potential member, if a suitable form that fills the needs of all is to be designed. Thus, for example, six major regional hospitals, concerned with their local competition and with the desire to compete with the for-profits, wanted to determine some form of association that would enable them to start activities of joint interest but would also leave them free to compete in their local areas. Competitive analysis revealed a list of capabilities which was used to determine potential activities (based upon existing capacity) that would complement identified needs. The structure selected was an alliance in the form of a tiered holding company. Each member formed a holding company in its own area, enabling it to acquire local organizations or to start services for them. A "super" holding company was then formed, held by the six members, to provide corporate services (e.g., planning and feasibility studies), and to hold joint venture corporations for each of the new activities (Figure 5-11). These new activities were then available to the members themselves, or, through their own holding company as local franchises, to their local service area(s).

It cannot be emphasized too strongly that form should follow function, and the structure of a collaborative enterprise should be dictated by the likely activities that will be carried out. Of course, some format is required to get to the point of deciding on activities—and if there are no activities to be seriously considered, then there should be no collaboration. Moreover, the structure should alter as the activities change and require structural adaptation.

Figure 5-11

Tiered Holding Company (Alliance)

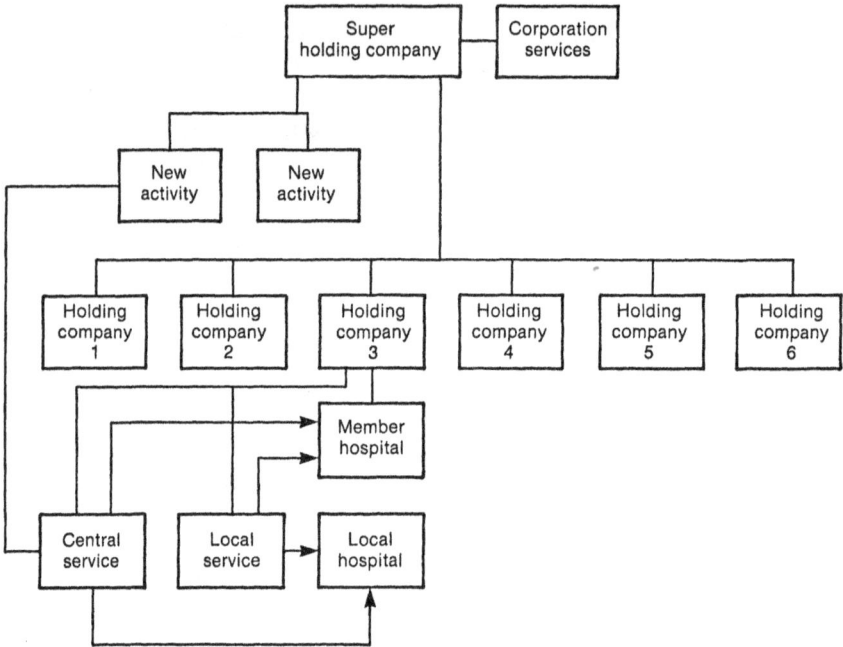

Collaboration and Paradigm Changes

Mark Twain reportedly said, "Even if you're on the right track you'll get run over if you just sit there." Throughout this chapter the need is stressed for managers to move aggressively in exploring areas where collaborative behavior may reduce levels of uncertainty and resource constraint—managers must never sit on the track and wait to be run over. However, it should be clear from the many factors, checklists, and issues discussed in this chapter that entering and successfully maintaining collaborative arrangements—especially those where some loss of autonomy is required—can be an extensive and difficult change for any organization.

Too much change can be overwhelming. Managers and their staffs must be anchored in stability and security to entertain change without becoming unhinged; ironically, however, anchors are usually found in the fabric of the organization's culture, which itself must evolve and adapt to accommodate the demands of changes elsewhere in the organization. Collaboration may represent a major, multidimensional (paradigmatic) alteration in an organization, a radical shift from the traditions of autonomy and self-determination. Managers must sequence and modulate this change process for staff. The process of modulating the intraorganizational behavioral and attitudinal changes needed to accompany (complement) the demands of collaboration represent a paradigmatic change, a concept which was introduced in Chapter 1.

Summary

The idea of collaboration is too often seductive. Collaboration should only be pursued by health care delivery institutions as a means of furthering their competitive strategy. In that respect, collaboration affords the opportunity to enter a market or to aggregate resources.

When considering collaboration, failure to assess the match between potential collaborators can impose a heavy penalty in failure or delay, with concurrent costs. Collaboration is rarely "pure." Often institutions may choose to collaborate while continuing to compete in some areas. Any collaborative form must therefore take into account both the desire to collaborate and the continuation of competition.

Three sets of factors are important: the first describes whether or not there is indeed a rationale for joint activity; the second delineates the significant forces for and against collaboration; and the third indicates the compatibility of institutional styles, which may become a problematic issue.

The period during which a collaborative venture is being considered may be extremely sensitive, since key staff may be lost to other institutions because of rumors and speculation.

Once collaboration is entered into, to proceed effectively, certain critical tasks must be accomplished in a series of stages: (1) a delineation of purpose, (2) assessment of appropriate membership, (3) institution of effective decision-making mechanisms, and (4) the determination of activities that are meaningful and nonthreatening. These tasks must be addressed thoroughly and iteratively.

Finally, a variety of structural forms are possible, each of which may be more or less appropriate to different sets of activities and different stages of the collaborative process. Collaborating institutions should periodically reexamine their structures to determine whether the structures are still appropriate to the evolving set of common activities in which the institutions engage.

Restructuring

*Half the failures in life arise from pulling in
one's horse as he is leaving.*
J. C. and A. W. Hare

This chapter discusses restructuring and unbundling and describes the situation in which an organization may want to restructure, considering the main issues, risks, and advantages.

What Are Restructuring and Unbundling?

As discussed in Chapter 2, there are four major strategies (apart from maintaining the status quo) which managers can adopt as they respond to the challenge of change: (1) focus or specialization in several services and products; (2) development of vertically integrated systems, i.e., mini-health-systems, which can be achieved by acquiring different types of health units and providing a range of services; (3) product/service diversification, and/or (4) differentiation. Various positioning activities are needed to move towards any one of these strategies.

Restructuring This is one such positioning activity. By definition, restructuring is an organizational realignment; however, it may be directed

116

towards the organization's administrative operations, clinical services, or fiscal structure. Restructuring should never be undertaken for its own sake, but should be directed towards one or more of the following outcomes:

Financial improvement.
Better management.
Expansion in one or more service directions or markets.
Tax advantages.
Regulatory advantages.

The term restructuring is a general one, broad enough to include such activities as increasing or collapsing the number of departments/units, adding a layer (layers) to an organization's clinical or administrative hierarchy, or changing the fiscal management of the organization. More importantly, restructuring is a process that allows managers and staff to think differently about what they provide and how they provide it. Restructuring should follow redirection of strategy, but, like other positioning activities, the act may precede its articulation, making redirection of strategy more possible. However, be guided by at least a sense of strategic direction.

Unbundling This is a specific type of restructuring activity: activities once grouped together are now separated. For example, activities which used to exist within departments of a hospital would now be suffused with sufficient resources to become separate divisions or even independent corporate businesses. Free of the institution, the activities can respond to the needs of the marketplace, can be contracted to new institutions, or can even be contracted back to the original institution (e.g., offering services for a fee instead of carrying them out under a departmental budget). By comparison, general organizational restructuring need not involve the physical separation of activities from or within the organization. In many instances, following restructuring, the realigned activities still fall under the managerial roof of the institution, clustered into departments that dictate policy, control financial plans, etc. In unbundling, however, the institution creates an autonomous, aggressive growth stock.

It is possible that in some instances unbundling may be simply a separation of hospital activities into distinctly managed divisions; most often, however, it involves setting up a series of separately incorporated corporations, some for-profit, some not-for-profit, under an umbrella corporation. Services or activities are removed from the "protection" of the organization to become a subsidiary business. Like any other entrepreneurial venture, these may succeed gloriously or fail to thrive. The basic principles of unbundling, then, are as follows:

Separation of the activity from the parent organization (or at least from other similar activities).
Different organizational structure.
Different strategic management.

A recently emerging principle of business organization calls these "unbundled" activities *strategic business units* (SBUs). In the health field an equivalent term, *strategic service units* (SSUs) may be more appropriate. The use of strategic business units began in 1971 in the executive offices of General Electric, the world's most diversified company. As it evolved, the SBU concept of planning followed several principles:

> The diversified firm should be managed as a "portfolio" of businesses, with each business serving a clearly defined product market segment with a clearly defined strategy.
>
> Each business unit in the portfolio should develop a strategy tailored to its capabilities and competitive needs but consistent with the overall corporate capabilities and needs.
>
> The total portfolio of businesses should be managed by allocating capital and managerial resources to serve the interests of the firm as a whole to achieve balanced growth in sales, earnings, and asset mix at an acceptable and controlled level of risk. In essence, the portfolio should be designed and managed to achieve an overall corporate strategy.[1]

The principle of the strategic service unit (SSU) in health care organizations is similar. It helps management identify distinct markets which require different kinds of strategic actions, and it also differentiates activities simply requiring maintenance effort from those calling for aggressive administrative and financial investment. Generally, activities grouped in an SSU must share one or more of: customers, markets, competition, or mission.[2]

When to Consider Creating SSUs

Managers may consider the creation of SSUs (unbundling one or more services) for various purposes. In the case of diversification, unbundling frees a potentially profitable service from departmental policies, organizational overhead rates, and institutional marketing approaches, to develop a greater market potential. If managers believe that a healthy market exists for a selected service, and, further, that the full market potential for that service is thwarted by the need to conform to the policies of the

---

[1]William K. Hall, "SBUs: Hot New Topic in the Management of Diversification," *Business Horizons*, February 1978, 21, pp. 17-25.

[2]"Conversation with Reginald H. Jones and Frank Doyle," *Organizational Dynamics*, Winter 1982, pp. 42-63.

broader organization, then unbundling may be a wise strategic choice. For example, a hospital may set up its radiology laboratory as an SSU. By doing so, the laboratory can serve not only the hospital's need for radiological services but can also market services to clinics, group practices, and other hospitals in the area.

A second situation in which managers may want to consider unbundling is the case where this strategy would increase revenues. For example, Blue Cross and Medicare often reimburse providers at different rates for the same services. By spinning off an independent business entity, an organization may avoid reimbursement differentials which are linked to provider type. The Health Corporation of the Archdiocese of Newark (HCAN) provides an example of organizational restructuring. HCAN is an umbrella health corporation which was established in 1981 to manage and govern St. James Hospital of Newark, St. Michael's Medical Center of Newark, and St. Mary's Hospital of Orange, as well as Roman Catholic health programs, services, and facilities within the Archdiocese of Newark. Proposed restructuring (Figure 6-1) is intended to bring in other Catholic hospitals under the umbrella corporation, as well as to facilitate engaging in a variety of new administrative and medical services. The purpose of organizational restructuring is to *gain the maximum possible financial benefits both in the capital market and in streaming cash flows* from a possible new variety of services and institutions, as well as to maximize organizational flexibility.

In addition to removing a service from the overhead of an institution and increasing its revenue-generating potential, setting up an SSU (unbundling) may provide another kind of advantage: an easing of regulatory constraints. For example, in some states, radiology labs can operate under the regulatory guidelines for radiology corporations, rather than under guidelines which apply to health care institutions, thereby giving the service wider latitude.

Fourth, unbundling a service may increase the volume of business for that service. Increased volume, in turn, affords a greater management and fiscal management capacity, which then can lead to contracting out management services and to consulting.

In short, unbundling—in the right circumstances—removes a service from an organizational cul de sac. It produces dividends (a greater volume of business) which produce further dividends (improved management and fiscal management) and services which can be offered through contracting and consulting.

When Is Unbundling Likely to Be Successful?

An unbundling venture, to be successful, must meet two sets of organizational needs. First, it must satisfy the parent institution's need for

Figure 6-1

Proposed Corporate Structure

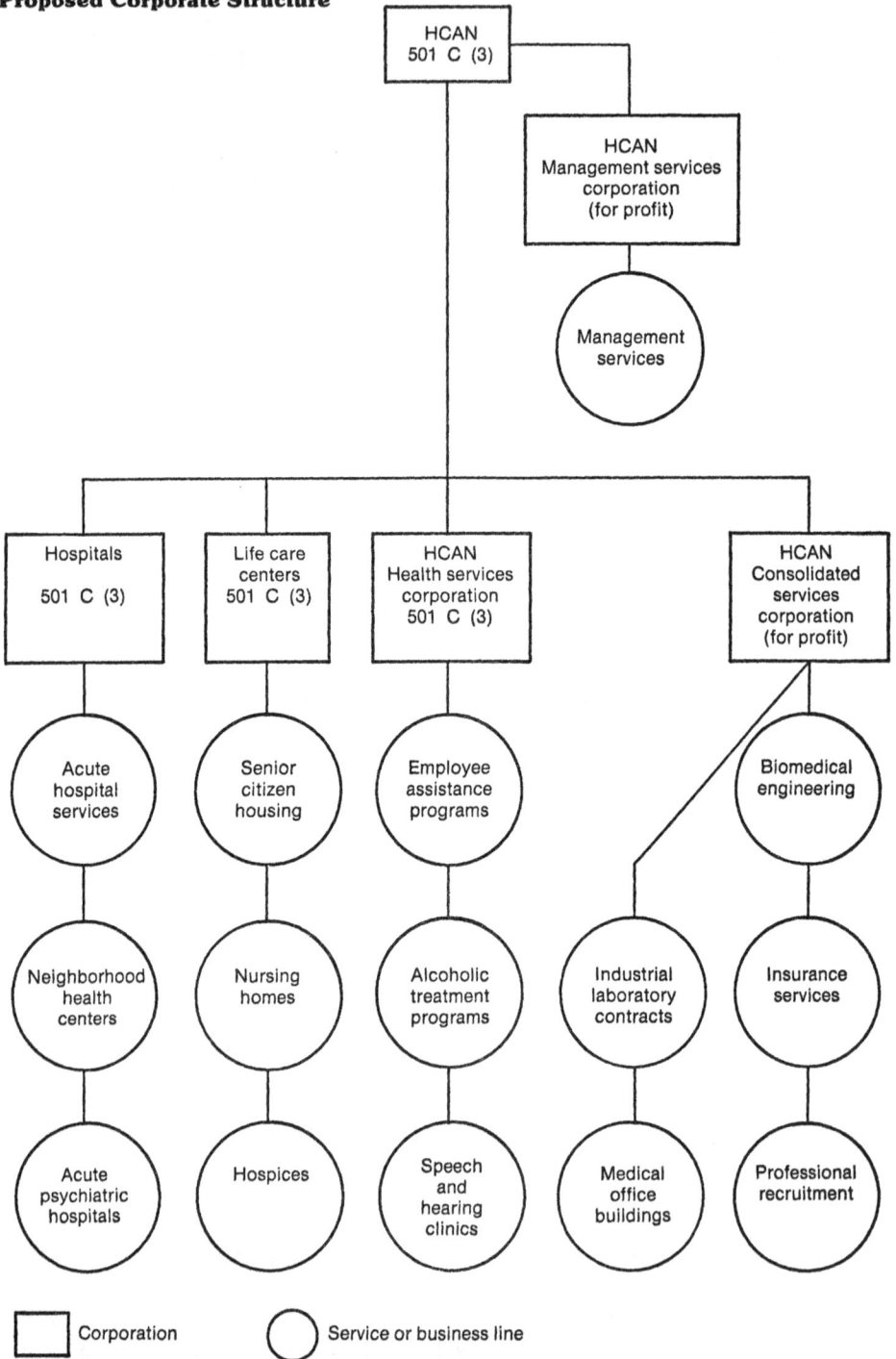

- HCAN 501 C (3)
- HCAN Management services corporation (for profit)
  - Management services
- Hospitals 501 C (3)
  - Acute hospital services
  - Neighborhood health centers
  - Acute psychiatric hospitals
- Life care centers 501 C (3)
  - Senior citizen housing
  - Nursing homes
  - Hospices
- HCAN Health services corporation 501 C (3)
  - Employee assistance programs
  - Alcoholic treatment programs
  - Speech and hearing clinics
- HCAN Consolidated services corporation (for profit)
  - Industrial laboratory contracts
  - Medical office buildings
  - Biomedical engineering
  - Insurance services
  - Professional recruitment

☐ Corporation   ◯ Service or business line

corporate control. Obviously, a hospital does not want to spin off its radiology service to reap a greater profit unless a share of those profits accrue to the parent. Nor would it want to set up a subsidiary that would compete with services still controlled by or housed within the parent. Therefore, the parent institution must ensure that it has some majority ownership in this new growth stock. The institution wants to see the subsidiary do well—do better than it could if the service remained unbundled—and it wants to reap some benefits from the subsidiary's success.

Second, there are organizational needs of the new subsidiary to consider: the new SSU must have a sufficient degree of autonomy. Since the new entity will bear the brunt of failures that occur, its leadership will want the authority to carry out management and marketing strategies necessary for achieving success. New leadership is likely to want a staff distinct from the staff of the parent institution. These managers also need to be free from financial constraints—the overhead allocation which would be borne as a department—and also from external management constraints. The spin-off organization needs to have both more money and more management muscle.

In the process of assessing the chances for a successful subsidiary, there are several key issues which the parent institution and the new enterprise must each address. For the institution, the key questions are how much the new subsidiary can serve the short- and long-term needs of the parent—in terms of income, unearthing new markets, bringing in allied business, and strengthening the institution's hand as a health care provider. For the new SSU, the focus is on accurately costing what it offers: charging appropriately and assessing start-up costs, potential markets, and client needs.

For both the parent and the new group, there is the key question of staff and management style. Rapidly growing SSUs need managers who are entrepreneurial types, very different from the more stable and reactive people who can successfully oversee steady, established, unspectacular services. The parent group faces the task of finding the appropriate people to manage a new and aggressive SSU. Both groups face the task of integrating very different management styles into the overall corporate force. Notably the corporate staff of the parent institution may change as a result of spinning off the new subsidiary.

The size of the new venture should be a function of management style as much as business volume. Size reflects the personality of the CEO and the degree of control he or she wants to exert. It also reflects the texture of the relations between the parent and the subsidiary. If the newly formed subsidiary is going to be entirely independent in its marketing and operating strategy, and linked to the parent only through finances and control systems, the corporate staff will be smaller. If the subsidiary is still being guided in its day-to-day operations by the parent institution, the parent will continue to provide many centralized services to its subsidiaries as a way of maintaining control. The corporate staff required in this case will be larger.

Managing the Mix

As an institution surveys its clinical and management services to determine what aspects might profitably be unbundled, it must ask "which" and "how many"?

Unbundling may set up an SSU that offers diagnostic services, physical therapy, radiation, or laboratory or cardio-pulmonary testing. Any one of these, previously a medical department in a hospital, may become an independent group, doing business by contracting with the parent and with other health groups needing its services. Any one of these may be a likely candidate for unbundling, as may all of them together. Ultimately, an institution may wind up with a series of service groups, all linked to the institution by contract instead of by organizational hierarchy.

A wide range of management services—administrative, marketing, planning—can also be unbundled, one at a time or all together, depending on the specific service's potential to stand alone. Shared services, such as laundry or joint purchasing, can become the function of a subsidiary, contracted to the parent institution and to other health care groups. Real estate, rather than a management or medical service, can also form the basis of a subsidiary. For example, a company can be incorporated that owns the land on which a hospital is located. This company may own other land as well, leasing it to tenants.

Figure 6-2 shows examples of the range of services that can be unbundled into free-standing SSUs. In assessing the best mix, it is necessary to look beyond the immediate geographic community to a wider area, to see what the marketplace might be for a particular product or service-based group. In the case of an expanding HMO, geography may become an obstacle. If the HMO has expanded from one center to several and has acquired a hospital, then it is common for all to report to a corporate headquarters. But as the plan expands and additional centers are added, the distance between new centers and the hospital may become an obstacle. At that point, the HMO will have to decide whether to (1) acquire or build a second hospital; (2) restructure on a different geographic basis; or (3) maintain its present arrangement and risk a drop in patient enrollment because hospitalization may be relatively inaccessible to some patients.

Because the reality of a present structure is often so compelling that it is difficult for an institution to even consider future alternatives, there is an automatic theoretical advantage to thinking of restructuring and unbundling. In the case of the HMO above, for example, the focus on compre-

Figure 6-2

Services Which Might Be Unbundled into Free-Standing Strategic Service Units (SSUs)

Laboratory	Long-term care and skilled nursing
Equipment repair	Equipment purchasing/leasing
Cardio-pulmonary testing	Out-patient services
Strategic planning and design	Organizational management
Dietary services	Real estate
Respiratory therapy	Group purchasing
Renal dialysis	Biomedical engineering
Radiology	Legal consultation
Physician/nurse recruiting	Public relations
Computer tomographic services	Fund development
Physical therapy	Miscellaneous consulting
Data processing	Consulting in specialized clinical services
Medical records services	Emergency medical services

hensive, local market centers restricts thinking about redefining the business to include, for example, supplying employee care in industrial plants.

A number of models for unbundling currently exist nationwide.[3] Two for-profit ones are briefly described below:

American Medical International (AMI) has formed a broad range of subsidiaries which service the parent organization as well as others:

Subsidiary	Service Provided
American Clinical Labs	A reference lab
AMI Technical Engineering	Repairs of high-tech equipment
Cardio Dynamic Labs	Cardio-pulmonary function testing
Friesen International	Hospital strategic planning and design
Hyatt Medical Food Service	Sells dietary services
Hyatt Medical Management	Sells total arrangement
Inhalation Therapy Services	Respiratory therapy services
Medical Career Services	Physician recruiting
Mobile C. T. Services	Sells computer tomographic service
National Therapy Associates	Physical therapy
Pharmaceuticals Management	Manages hospital pharmacies
Physical Therapy Associates	Out-patient physical therapy
Professional Services	Data-processing management
Stat Records	Medical records services
Stewart Design	Architectural services

National Medical Enterprises (NME) has numerous subsidiaries. Some of the most active in selling services to the health industry are:

---

[3]Much of this information was supplied by Rick Blume, of Blythe Eastman Payne Webber Health Care Funding Inc., to whom I am very grateful.

Subsidiary	Service Provided
Implementation Mastro Planning	Planning services
Millhaven	Drugstores, long-term care, and skilled nursing
International Medical Enterprises	International hospital management
Metro Hospital Supply	Equipment purchasing service
National Funding	Equipment leasing and financing
National Medical Oxygen DBA (Livingston Medical Products)	Sells medical gases
Syndicated Office Systems	Sells business offices and out-patient services
Stolte	Design and construction
TAD Avanti	Phone answering devices and services
Medical Ambulatory Care	Out-patient services

It is interesting to note that the subsidiary activities of NME accounted for 39 percent of total revenue and 24 percent of income before interest and taxes. Clearly, these diversified activities are important to the health-care-provider aspects of these two investor-owned companies.

Three non-profit organizations are also described, which very much follow the pattern of the for-profits.

Health Central (HC) is an example of diversification in the nonprofit sector. HC is presently a single corporation which owns or manages 19 hospitals and nursing homes and is affiliated with 178 additional facilities. Services sold to affiliates and non-member hospitals include:

Administration	Education
Financial management	Clinical development
Planning	Consultation
Data processing	Emergency services
Personnel recruitment	Fund development
Group purchasing	Legal consultation

The corporation does have one subsidiary, a real estate holding company called Twenty Eight-Ten Inc. This subsidiary also serves as an insurance company for the corporation, handling worker's compensation and general liability insurance.

Baylor University Medical Center, another nonprofit which owns or manages five acute care hospitals, has also diversified. In addition to running hospitals it owns the following companies:

Subsidiary	Service Provided
Gilmer Convalescent and Nursing Center	Skilled nursing facility
Baylor Medical Plaza Inn	Medical Office Building
Gaston Construction Company	Constructs hospitals and has limited outside activity
Church University Insurance Company	Captive insurance company

Lutheran General Hospital is also a nonprofit that has restructured by setting up two holding companies. The structure separates provider from nonprovider activities. The provider activities include the hospital and an alcoholism treatment center. The nonprovider holding company governs a corporation that provides many activities which the hospital has traditionally performed, for example, pastoral counseling, psychiatry, and services for the aged. Additionally, Lutheran General governs a for-profit consulting and management contract firm. A foundation is also separately incorporated which acts as a conduit between the two holding companies and performs traditional fund-raising activities.

To explain why all of these nonprofit systems are analogous to the investor-owned organizations described earlier, it may help to examine a simplified model. For example, a unit hospital operating as a nonprofit corporation would not realize a return on capital. Furthermore, if the hospital were taking in outside work to provide extra revenue, it would have experienced an allocation of overhead expense against those revenues to reduce Medicare costs. Both return on capital (on part of the hospital assets) and avoidance of the overhead allocation against the extra revenue base can be avoided by a change in the corporate structure.

If, on the other hand, the unit hospital were owned by a parent company which also had a foundation or other nonprovider subsidiary, the subsidiary could invest in a taxable, ancillary health care service company. The ancillary health care service company could purchase the lab assets, for example, from the nonprofit provider, and subsequently sell lab service back to the nonprofit provider. As a for-profit corporation, the services sold could include a return on capital (profit factor) and would not be subjected to random allocation of overhead by Medicare. This configuration is diagramed in Figure 6-3.

Figure 6-3

Simplified Restructuring Model

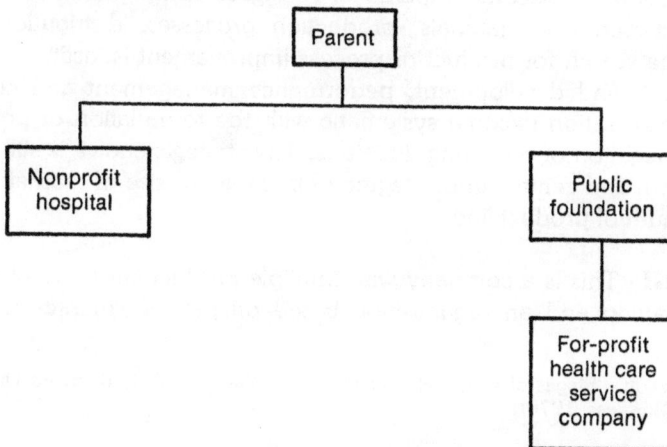

There is an advantage in having the capacity to sell health care in these unbundled units. Change in corporate structure may combat difficult aspects of regulations. The most important advantage, however, is the ability to successfully meet the forthcoming competition within the health care providers industry. Competition is coming in several ways. One, the marketplace is basically overbuilt, which by itself should create competition. Two, the current administration is seeking ways to limit the rising costs for Medicare and Medicaid.

Strategic service units will enable services to be sold competitively in larger volume, to be sold outside the hospital, and to be sold with an appropriate margin, yet at lower cost than the hospital could afford to charge by itself.

Corporate Development and Restructuring

When is it appropriate for an institution to pursue restructuring? This can be partially answered by reviewing previous work on the stages of corporate development and by making comparisons between corporate development in general and that of health institutions in particular.[4]

One model characterizes each stage of corporate development by the way a firm is managed and by the scope of strategic choice available to it.

Stage I   This stage represents a single-product (or line of products) company with little or no formal structure. The firm is run by the owner, who personally performs most of the managerial functions, using subjective and unsystematic measures of performance, reward, and control. The strategy of this form is what the owner-manager wants it to be.

Stage II   This is the single-product firm grown so large that functional specialization has become imperative. A degree of integration has developed between raw materials, production processes, distribution, and sales. The search for product or process improvement is institutionalized in research and development; performance management and control, and compensation become systematic with the formulation of policy to guide delegation of operating decisions. The strategic choice is still under top control and centers upon degree of integration, size of market share, and breadth of product line.

Stage III   This is a company with multiple product lines and channels of distribution and an organization based on product/market relation-

---

[4]B. R. Scott, "Stages of Corporate Development, Parts I and II" (Harvard University School of Business, 1970).

ships rather than function. Its businesses are not to a significant degree integrated; they have their own markets. Its research and development is oriented to new products rather than improvements and its measurement and control systems are increasingly systematic and oriented to results. Strategic alternatives are phrased in terms of entry into and exit from industries, allocation of resources by industry, and rate of growth.

As an organization grows, it may pass from Stage I through Stage II and into Stage III. As it does so, the range of strategies available to it will also grow in complexity. As companies diversify, the definitions of their "business" turn away from literal description of products and markets toward general statements about product lines and marketing objectives. A conglomerate firm made up of many different businesses will need to have many different strategies, perhaps one for each of its individual lines of products and services.

This model of the organizational stages of development is useful for managers of health care organizations who are weighing different kinds of strategies. In particular, it offers managers a framework for looking at their organization to determine whether its size, diversification of services, or other factors merit organizational restructuring, or whether continuance of the existing structure is in order.

A good example of this is Nursing Homes Associated (NHA). Founded in 1970, NHA has as its goal providing total care to the elderly. The concept behind NHA is to provide this care in a stratified, pyramidal structure: the sophisticated, skilled care of the acute general care hospital is the top level; skilled nursing homes constitute the middle strata; and homes for the elderly, out-patient facilities, and support services form the base.

Up until 1980, the organizational structure, which had grouped like institutions together into divisions, e.g., nursing home division, old age home division, had worked quite well, and NHA had grown and developed. However, as NHA's clientele widened and the demand for care increased, there was a question of how to balance the need for individual autonomy in the various institutions with the need for central coordination by the NHA administration. Moreover, it was becoming clear that nonmedical services for the elderly were becoming an increasingly important part of NHA's product line.

With respect to the issue of restructuring, NHA is an example of an organization which might consider diversification into nonmedical services that could be provided to its clients as well as marketed outside. Other issues concern the need to create a centralized corporate administrative office to oversee the activities of individual institutions. How large should this office be? What skills are needed for its staff? The answer to both of these questions depends on the goal of NHA: does the organization have as its goal growth, improved operating efficiency, or consulting to its internal members? Moreover, is the present organizational structure appropriate given that NHA is now providing a total range of care for the elderly in its geographic area? Should NHA pursue a single organizational strategy, or is it now a Stage II or Stage III firm where multiple strategies are more appropriate? If so, should the old age homes division go off in a different direction? Or should a mini-regional structure be developed in which each mini-region has one set of institutions (e.g., old age home, nursing home, etc.) in which cross-referral takes place.

Using NHA as an example, it can be seen that restructuring is generally not an issue for an organization in Stage I, where there is only one main product. However, as organizations grow larger and offer multiple products, restructuring can improve the efficiency and effectiveness with which the organization operates. The basic issue in the later stages of growth is how differentiation and integration are to take place. What makes sense at one stage may not at another. Like institutions (old age homes, nursing homes) do require similar skills in management. But the critical issues for the enterprise may change, and what must be different (differentiation) alters. Larger organizations with more complex functions require more effective integrative mechanisms. Centralized planning and control, therefore, may become more important. The reverse side of the coin for unbundling into distinct enterprises is a need for very effective central coordination and control of the new, diverse activities.

Given the establishment of these controls, one of the real advantages of unbundling is that it offers further possibilities for product specialization and for removing the constraints that organizational structure places on products which may be marketed more effectively as autonomous lines of business. By the time an organization (for example, a very large hospital) has reached Stage III, serious attention to organizational restructuring as a positioning activity is not only desirable—it is imperative.

In summary, restructuring is a positioning activity which frees managers to pursue strategic moves which might otherwise be constrained by their institution's structure. Unbundling is a particular form of restructuring in which activities once grouped together are separated out and perhaps actually "spun off" into autonomous business ventures. The phenomenon of unbundling first began in the area of shared services, involving such mundane activities as laundry, purchasing, and the pharmacy.

Restructuring and unbundling mean that it is no longer possible to consider competition as occurring only between health care organizations in a defined geographic area. Unbundling frees activities from the geographic confines of a single town or region. The unbundling process, together with the product market analysis discussed in Chapter 4, have enabled managers to recognize that services once contained within their organizations as clinical divisions (or operations) can be separated out in a fashion that is at once responsive to patient needs and profitable.

The basic and underlying concept is separating like from unlike activities, and the recognition that managing different activities effectively requires alternative resource inputs, marketing strategies, administrative acumen, and strategic action. While this process may be initially easier to identify for administrative services, certain clinical services are also amenable to unbundling.

Unbundling is a trend which has only recently emerged, but the competitive pressures which face health care organizations will undoubtedly make it more common. The health system of the future will probably take the form of one of two different organizations, both based to some degree on the SSU principle. In one type of organization, much allied to the industrial conglomerate, groups of hospitals collaborate and then reorganize into distinct businesses along SSU lines. Each of these distinct businesses, whether administrative—providing management services—or clinical, will direct its energy outward to a non-geographically defined service market.

The second model is that of the mini-health-system. Rather than expanding into unconstrained service markets in an aggressive fashion, this model attempts to capture patients within designated markets by offering them all possible modalities of care within a single, integrated system. The SSU principle will enable such systems to function more effectively. The only limitation to this form of organization may lie in the possibility of changes in laws governing restraint of trade; however, such legal action is unlikely to be instituted by the federal government. More likely, unsuccessful competitors with organizations which have formed mini-health-systems will raise legal concern over monopolistic practices.

Summary

In this book, the term *restructuring* is used more broadly than often is the case in the literature. As resources are addressed more accurately to product market segments, and as resources are aggregated, it becomes important for organizations to rethink how their resources are grouped. Traditionally, health care organizations have tended to organize along the lines dictated by demography or disease. However, different product market segments require different strategies, and those segments with similar strategies may be grouped together in what are called strategic service units (SSUs). Beyond the individual institution, as multi-institutional systems develop, activities with similar strategies may be grouped together through corporate restructuring. While some early corporate restructuring was dictated by regulatory factors, restructuring in the broadest sense directs activities more effectively toward markets but requires a difference in managerial style.

Managing the Physician | CHAPTER 7

Physicians are like kings—
They brook no contradiction.

John Webster

Previous chapters have addressed organizational issues pertaining to competitive strategy. Here, issues concerning the role of physicians vis-à-vis organizational strategy and strategic management will be discussed under the following rubrics:

A brief history of institutional-physician relationships.

The physicians' role in institutional governance and strategy.

The physician as supplier and marketer of medical services.

The physician in institutional strategy.

The role of the physician in institutional strategy development and implementation is critical. Despite the best efforts of managers to position their organizations effectively, competitive strategy cannot be implemented without supportive and appropriate behavioral responses from the primary provider of medical care—the physician. Thus far, the discussion in this book has focused on those forces affecting competitive organizations. Physician behavior, however, responds to still other forces, including income, prestige, desire to practice medicine in compliance with the physician's perceptions of what constitutes good clinical care, and a reasonable mix between income-producing and leisure time. The challenge to managers is to bring the interests—or at least the behaviors—of physicians into line with the strategic needs of the institution. More often than not, this will require thoughtful and systematic manipulation of the forces which drive physicians' attitudes and behavior.

The basic issue facing administrators is that physicians are given proprietary claim over the "proper application of medical care" in general, the types of "products" and "services" through which care should be rendered, and the amounts and types of care that particular consumers (ought to) demand and physicians (ought to) supply. Freidson uses the term "professional dominance" to characterize the consumer-demand and provider-supply defining authority of physicians as a group.[1] These authorities/capacities are reflected in three major roles which physicians play in relation to health care organizations:

Governance—the influence of physicians on organizational policies and administration.

Operations—physicians in their roles as providers of care, sources of patient referrals to the organization, and transformers of medical resources.

Strategy—the influence of physicians on organizational goals and strategy, as well as the way in which strategy influences physician behavior and attitudes.

A brief survey of these roles will serve as an introduction to this chapter's main focus: a detailed discussion of how physicians' roles interact with and affect various strategic and positioning activities.

More often than not, health care institutions have been appendages of physicians' medical practices; however, it must be acknowledged that there is variation in the extent to which institutional policies and procedures are controlled by the physicians who use institutions as a place in which to treat and/or provide beds for their patients. For example, proprietary hospitals—owned privately and run for profit—are devoted to providing services that only physicians are licensed to give. Insofar as physicians are the gatekeepers who determine which and how many patients are hospitalized, and decide what shall be done to treat them, it follows that whether or not physicians own the proprietary hospitals (as is fairly common), the hospital's policies are frequently focused on accommodating the needs and desires of the physicians. This posture may be tempered somewhat by the demands of patients, the economics of reimbursement, and other requisites of profit-making behavior. The physician

---

[1] E. Freidson, *Profession of Medicine* (New York: Dodd, Mead, 1971).

who brings to the institution the most patients or the best-paying patients will have the greatest influence on policy; and policy in general will be reflective of a laissez-faire attitude: the physician will be free to do more or less what she or he pleases medically, with little or no supervision of medical performance other than by a group of peers. By comparison, within voluntary and community hospitals, much of the control of hospital policy has been passing out of the hands of physicians and into the hands of boards that "own," and administrative staffs that manage, the institution. Policy has become divided into several spheres, with medical staff controlling much of the policy specifically related to their work and administrative staff controlling the day-to-day affairs of the hospital.

In organizations other than hospitals, the governing strength of the physician also varies. A group practice is physician owned and dominated. An Independent Practice Association (IPA) is physician owned and dominated, but has to be responsive to the performance characteristics of its members, possibly sanctioning undesirable behavior on the part of a few to maintain the best interests of the entire association. The relationship between the IPA and the physician is, however, different than the relationship in an HMO, where a physician is a salaried employee. Group practices, HMOs, and hospitals which salary physicians have a different opportunity to influence physicians than do those organizations in which the physician is reimbursed on a fee-for-service basis. Where physicians have alternative sites at which to practice, the influence that can be brought to bear upon them—and their effects on governance and operations—is different.

Physicians also tend to influence institutional strategy. For example, within organizations which have the narrow aim of "servicing" physician demand for beds, strategy is closely tied to the needs and interests of the physician. For other types of institutions that include nonmedical as well as non-physician-dominated goals in their strategic definition, there may be greater imposition of rules on physician behavior. Clearly, however, the role of the physician vis-à-vis organizational strategy must be carefully considered. For one thing, physicians tend to become very concerned when hospitals engage in diversification strategies because they feel that the hospital's energy and resources are being directed away from patient care. As the interests and practice patterns of physicians diverge from the needs and interests of health care institutions, there are three possible outcomes:

1. They may separate from the institution and develop their own enterprises to a greater degree.
2. They may attempt to enter more aggressively into the management of the health care institution and thus modulate the impact of changes in institutional behavior/goals.

3. The managers of health institutions may develop (possibly with the input of physicians) incentives which would make it attractive for physicians to bring their practice patterns and behaviors in line with changes in the organization's strategy/goals/behaviors.

Where physicians (as groups) become distinct entities and change the nature of their affiliations with health care organizations, they clearly become a competitive force to be reckoned with in many of the ways thus far described in this book. Some physician groups may not only "reform" themselves as separate entities outside of organizations, but may also hire their own staff and equipment, compete directly with existing institutions, and even shift demand for services from one institution to another, affecting all institutions' competitive positions.

As a response to this potential threat, there is a new shift away from using the physician as the primary "marketing" force to provide patients for health care institutions. Instead, many institutions are marketing their own services to patients or marketing themselves to physicians by attracting the physician with favorable conditions and resources. For example, St. James Hospital in Newark has adopted a strategy of moving into occupational health services, thus attracting a local commercial market. The hospital's intent is also to create a service base and an environment which will attract physicians interested in occupational medicine.

In short, the physician plays an important, but mixed, role in organizational behavior and strategic options. In his or her role as major arbiter of health care resources, case mix, and costs, the physician can be a major force in governance, operations/marketing, and strategy formation/implementation. Managing the physician is clearly a crucial task for managers searching for new service markets and for ways of maximizing return on organizational investments through patient reimbursement.

Before turning to a more detailed discussion of physician roles and physician management, it is important to place the relationship of physicians and health care organizations—especially the hospital—in historical context and perspective. This overview provides a good background for understanding how the role of the physician has evolved and changed, as has the need to effectively "manage" physician behavior.

Physician-Institutional Relationships: A Brief History of the Issues

Physician behavior is a complex tapestry of professional (including personal, cognitive, peer-related, and ethical), and financial considerations. Essentially, there have been three distinct phases in the relationship between the administration of health care organizations and the physician.

During the first phase, physicians were either independent or agents of the administration, working for a paycheck and for some stability of practice. During the second phase, management began to be concerned about physician productivity. Management's response was to put pressure on the physicians, as well as (sometimes) to offer physicians incentives to become innovative and more productive in their patterns of practice. As management became increasingly directive of their activities, physicians shifted the nature of their relationship to the organization, feeling on some levels more identified with management but also more frustrated as they realized that management "called the shots" when it came to policy. More recently, both sides have been exploring ways in which the physician could become more a part of policymaking instead of an instrument of it. During the third phase, the relationship between institutional administrators and physicians has become far more complex and difficult as the result of rapid environmental changes and growing uncertainty. (Refer back to Chapter 1 for a discussion of these environmental changes.) Yet, the relationship between management and physicians is more critical than ever to the ability of health care organizations to serve the public adequately at an affordable price.

Latent Conflicts

Since early health care delivery organizations were essentially instruments of the physician, hospitals in particular were at his or her service. Cost and resource constraints were not an issue, so physicians essentially got their way. However, physician interests at that time generally coincided with those of the institutions, which grew, flourished, and become prestigious largely as a result of their physicians' activities. In the turbulent and uncertain environment of today and tomorrow, the behaviors and strategies which an institution has to adopt to survive and flourish may often be at odds with what the physician wishes to do in his or her practice of medicine. Physicians wish to retain control over their freedom to practice their craft. Managers, however have to pay attention to controlling costs and providing communities with whatever services they may need (versus those services the physician may want to provide). Moreover, regulatory programs, aimed at controlling costs, are, in fact, often targeted at institutional, not physician behavior. Thus, for example, the new Medicare reimbursement system limits payment to hospitals based upon standard variances for diagnosis-related groups (DRGs). Excess will not be reimbursed. The physician, however, has no direct limits on him or her; there is no inherent incentive in new Medicare policies for the physician to avoid keeping the patient in a health care institution as long as he or she sees fit or to use ancillaries efficiently. Rather, it is the hospital which will not be reimbursed if a patient's length of stay or consumption of ancillaries does not fall within standard limits. In other words, the institution must translate any limitations imposed by external regulatory policies into formal incentive or disincentive systems for physicians, who ultimately control resource utilization and allocation.

Two areas of conflict may result. First, any attempt to govern physicians' behavior will likely be seen to some degree as an encroachment upon autonomy and medical judgment. Moreover, an additional result of any attempt by management to reduce behaviors to "standards of care" may have a negative effect on physician incomes. This is both a systemwide (macro) and an institution-specific (micro) problem. The question is at what level should the remedy occur, and what remedy can be created that is likely to be effective? The macro-level incentives brought to bear on institutions (usually emanating from payment systems) must be translated into micro-level incentives, which are alternative approaches institutions may use to motivate physicians to be more cost conscious. A variety of incentives could be designed/identified, based on previous work in this area as well as on original thinking, so that managers might choose from a range of approaches those they feel would be most effective given their institution's internal composition, e.g., proportion of salaried physicians, institutionally based physicians, etc. Micro-level incentives need not be limited to financial incentives but may include provider education, peer review mechanisms, and other motivational tools such as case management conferences, discharge planning mechanisms, regular feedback on performance, peer support systems for efficient but "nontraditional" approaches to patient management, etc.

Many physicians have no prior experience in practicing medicine "efficiently." In addition, current structures of payment to providers have insulated physicians from the need to balance efficiency and quality of care concerns. At the micro level, the incentives to individual physicians should require that they now integrate these two concerns when making clinical decisions. Such programs for physicians should therefore be designed to give physicians both an orientation to cost-effective care and a mechanism for feedback on their performance. In particular, the feedback component of a program could be accomplished through peer review and conference formats.

The second area of conflict lies in the fact that there are clearly two types of variations from acceptable standards. One is the outlier, the other, and more important, the physician who exhibits only minor deviations in pattern of practice. Often this minor deviation is exhibited by physicians with high admission rates, which adds to an already significant problem. Because the deviation is minor, it is harder to do anything about (see below).

The potential for these conflicts between physicians and the administrators of health institutions has always existed and has long been recognized. Harris, for example, views the hospital as two firms, each with its own objectives, struggling over the allocation of resources.[2] Administrators wish to keep utiiization high and/or capacity low to ensure financial solvency. Physicians want to lower occupancy rates or increase capacity to ensure personal access to beds and ancillary services for their patients. Other authors have written about this issue, pointing out that hospital trustees often back physicians and increase the availability of high-technology services because these reflect well upon the hospital's image. Such authors generally believe that physicians run the hospital largely for their own convenience and at great expense and inefficiency. Regulatory practices, while punitive for the health institution overall, generally only punish the significant abuser where physicians are concerned. Little attention is paid to the smaller departure from acceptable standards, which is far more frequent, far harder to control, and far more damaging in its effects. If external regulators have had a difficult time taking on the physician, how much harder is it for the institutional manager when the physician controls so much of the destiny of the institution?

Consider an illustrative real example. In one teaching hospital, an analysis of two diagnosis-related groups (DRGs) showed that the same two physicians were responsible for most of the variance from standard. In DRG No. 165, simple pneumonia, these two physicians admitted 75 of the 110 cases (70 percent), jointly accounting for an average length of stay of 5.65 days per admission, as compared with the state average of 4.7 days. Only three physicians were responsible for a higher length of stay, and they accounted for only seven cases. In a second DRG, No. 169, bronchitis, these same two physicians accounted for 86 of 116 cases (74 percent), with an average length of stay of 4.7 days per admission, as compared with the state average of 3.7 days. These are clearly not abuses, since an average of one day longer per case does not constitute abuse. However, with the new DRG reimbursement system, the hospital employing these physicians may have difficulty getting paid for this extra day per person. What is the hospital manager to do about two physicians who together admit most of the case load in the hospital for these diseases?

The Conflicts Sharpen

The complexity and uncertainty of today's environment has sharpened these frequently dormant conflicts. Goldsmith feels, and practicing man-

---

[2]J. Harris, "The Internal Organization of Hospitals: Some Economic Implications," *Bell Journal of Economics*, no. 8 (1977), pp. 467–82.

agers certainly echo him, that the activities of today's hospital may compete directly with medical staff practices.[3] As the power of the manager has necessarily increased in institutions dealing with greater environmental complexity, the physician has begun to feel increasingly disenfranchised.

The conflict is not one between good and bad but is rather a genuine conflict of (differing) interests. Physicians are reasonably concerned about their incomes and reasonably concerned about doing what they believe to be best for their patients. They wish to design practices which will enable them to do what they like to do, what they have been trained to do and what is best for the kinds of patients they wish to treat. Managers of health organizations, on the other hand, are reasonably concerned with their revenues and with not going bankrupt. They have to deal with community pressures, competitive forces, and regulatory constraints. The problem for the physician is that in the past, it was possible to exert spasmodic control over the institution when circumstances seemed to call for it. The physicians' power and autonomy made this possible, despite the fact that most of the time it was not necessary. For physicians to control their destiny today, they have to have a far more consistent influence over many more issues. This represents an internal conflict for many physicians who would prefer to spend their time practicing medicine and not being managers, as well as a conflict between physicians and administrators.

The issue for the health manager is that physicians are still the primary suppliers of services (providers) and patients (marketers), and have major influence over the consumption of resources as well as the quality of patient-care activities. While it is true that the most difficult situation for the health manager is that of working with the fee-for-service practitioner as an independent, uncontrollable agent, the solution does not lie altogether in persuading physicians either to become full-time salaried employees or to form group practices with which the health manager then can negotiate. The reason is again simple but intractable: the behavioral incentives that cause physicians to behave in a fashion that is different from—and often at odds with—that of the health institution will remain the same, regardless of the nature of employment, as long as the control and incentive system does not significantly change.

The Physician and the Modern Hospital

Today's hospital is changing from a representative democracy in which some personnel were more equal than others, to a managed institution.

---

[3] J. C. Goldsmith, *Can Hospitals Survive? The New Competitive Health Care Market* (Homewood, Ill.: Dow Jones-Irwin, 1981).

The traditional structure, in which the medical staffs elected a president and a medical executive committee, essentially ensured that the attending physician's voice was heard without making too many administrative demands on the physician's clinical time. The health delivery organization of today has to attend to many constituencies, not just its physicians. In making decisions, managers must also move more rapidly. As a result, mechanisms that formerly worked quite effectively no longer do so. Physicians complain that decisions which affect them are made without their input. Managers feel that involving physicians in decision making blocks their activities or slows them down. The health field is in an extended transitional period in which health institutions are attempting to innovate organizational mechanisms that will be more effective tools for dealing with today's actualities. At the same time, physicians are struggling with their own evolving role in the health delivery organization. Should the doctor continue to be dominant in the medical model? Should he or she be a partner or merely a supplier of services with whom the institution negotiates? What is the appropriate role for the physician in governance, in strategy, and in operation? How can the institution control physician productivity, resource use, and quality, when these are so heavily influenced by the physician's actions? Should the physician become a manager or at least assume some managerial responsibilities? Will physicians willingly do this? If they do not wish to, then how can their voice appropriately be heard? Representation without responsibilities is no longer possible.

There are no neat separations or easy answers to these questions. The problem is not easy because many medical decisions have managerial consequences and vice versa. The problem is clearly not as simple as saying the "physicians are labor and management is management and the two must negotiate." What solutions may be viable? The remainder of this chapter will attempt to provide some preliminary responses to these issues.

The Physician in Governance

The key issue to be resolved is where to place checks and balances in the relationship between administration and physicians. The goal of achieving a system of governance in which there is an appropriate sharing of responsibility and power between management and physicians runs the danger of veering too much towards one of two extremes. The first is marked by a pattern in which institutions are run solely by management and physicians are hired as agents of management with little or no power and voice in decision making. The other extreme, one which some doctors might favor, is a total shift in which the board of the institution sets certain goals at the beginning of the year and the physicians run everything, including hiring whatever administrative help they need to carry out their wishes. Neither of these extremes is generally regarded as appropriate in a competitive environment.

One point to be kept in mind is that physicians are not a monolithic entity but are people with different interests and motivations. Some want control without responsibility, others are willing to assume responsibility, others simply wish to be left alone. As health organizations seek to determine and implement strategy, it is only too easy to characterize their physicians as a homogeneous block. Rarely, if ever, is this true. As management seeks to work with its physician staff, it has to recognize not only the formal entities that have been jointly created, but, also the range of views represented by individuals. Moreover, talking together—a solution often regarded as a panacea by managers, if not by physicians—is merely a first step which may allow the airing of concerns but not their resolution. It is probably accurate to state that the earlier stage of "representative democracy" in health institutions was analogous to that existing in Great Britain in the early part of the 20th century. While Britain had apparently been a democracy for centuries, the critical decisions influencing the country were, in fact, made by a small group of families who had held hereditary power for generations. Democracy existed more in form than in reality, and the empowering of a broad variety of constituencies brought this to life. True democracy means accepting "winning some" and "losing some." This is a state of sophistication arrived at by few countries, much less the health system of this nation.

The depth of the problem is brought home in the example of Doctor's Health Services (DHS), an Independent Practice Association that was created to compete with the perceived threat of a newly instituted Health Maintenance Organization. Formed by physicians in the interests of physicians, DHS was managed by a nonphysician. Initially DHS was successful, since the physicians who formed it were willing to accept some constraints in the face of an external competitive threat. The organization represented many dominant physician values such as the preservation of fee for service, the maintenance of health care delivery within the private sector, and the provision of comprehensive HMO benefits without change for the community physician. A major problem soon faced by DHS was a damaging increase in hospitalization rates. Some member physicians had become overutilizers. Simultaneously, however, other members were beginning to demand an absence of peer review or utilization controls, relaxation of reimbursement constraints, and a shutdown of attempts to control costs or modify referral patterns. In spite of their success—or indeed because of it—physicians were becoming self-indulgent. For the DHS administrator, the primary concern was to keep DHS's premium competitive and, in turn, control expense. Because of overutilization, costs had risen and the premium was up significantly. Good management in a financial sense was clearly beneficial, but the critical issue facing the manager of DHS was whether or not he could control the behavior of member physicians. The physicians set the policies, delivered care, and determined the fees. Their willingness to face the realities of life would ultimately determine whether DHS survived or went under.

A brief consideration of some additional examples is warranted. The merger that resulted in the formation of one major medical center in western Massachusetts, was negotiated by trustees and announced to administrators only one month before its inception and to physicians on the day of its being. This is perhaps the ultimate in noninvolvement of physicians in strategy; however, many managers feel that to involve physicians prematurely, if at all, in the determination of critical strategic issues is tantamount to making sure that that particular strategy is doomed to failure. Ken Mason, Chief Executive Officer of Midland Hospital, a small, 250-bed hospital discussed earlier, recognized that his general acute care facility could not continue to exist unchanged in a town with two larger competitive hospitals. He engaged in discussions with his counterparts at Johnston Memorial Hospital, and along with two key trustees from each institution, negotiated the outlines of a collaborative venture that resulted in a joint holding company to which both hospitals reported and which might eventually result in merger. It was only at this point that Mason involved Midland's medical executive committee, the president of the medical staff, and the vice president of medical affairs, in a session designed to present them with the realities of the hospital's strategic situation and the necessity for such collaboration. It is at least arguable that, if Mason had involved any physicians earlier, no such venture would have emerged. But the possibility of such a collaboration was in the air, and even in the relatively brief period in which it was felt that negotiations needed to go on without the involvement of physicians, some physicians did their best to transfer patients to other institutions, though they knew of nothing concrete to warrant such action. The result was to weaken Midland's bargaining position, though luckily not significantly. It is unclear whether earlier announcement would have avoided this, or precipitated a greater loss of admissions, since many of Midland's physicians had affiliations with each of the competitors.

Ted Jamison of the Health Corporation of the Archdiocese of Newark (HCAN) faced a similar issue of whether, when, and how to involve his physician staff in a key administrative decision. The medical school of Newark invited St. Michael, a 450-bed teaching hospital in the HCAN group, to join with another hospital in rebuilding on the medical campus adjacent to the medical school to increase the school's teaching capacity and programs. St. Michael's physicians recognized clearly that their interests would be hurt by such a move, and they made their concerns known. In this instance, their interests and those of St. Michael's management were consonant. HCAN strategy would also clearly be hurt by having its major hospital essentially captured by a rival group. Jamison chose to seek the advice of the St. Michael's physicians through a formal survey of their views about a variety of strategic options, including the one proposed. When the survey showed physician opinion to be nearly unanimous against the move, it provided compelling support for the CEO in his answer to the medical school's invitation.

At one time, many health managers kept their boards of trustees relatively ignorant of institutional activities, as a way of manipulating them. Today, it is generally recognized that a well-informed, highly educated, and capable board of trustees is an asset in strategy determination. Is this true for physicians?

Trustees are often relatively objective about the interests of their institutions; however, physicians are concerned not only about the welfare of the institution, but also about their personal interests. Moreover, physicians as a constituency of the institution are larger in number and more diverse in their concerns. If physicians are to be involved in strategy determination, there must be a formal involvement that will not bring this diversity into play and risk increasing uncertainty at critical moments. Some managers have a firm view that physicians should be involved in implementation but not determination of strategy. Others, especially in institutions with a forward-looking and sophisticated medical staff, prefer to involve physicians at the outset. Yet other managers selectively involve key individuals who they think may help the strategic process. As long as the interests of physicians remain divergent from those of the institution, institutional strategy determination involving the physician will be difficult. In such cases, which physicians should be involved must be a matter of administrative judgment, based upon the manager's perception of who will contribute to the process and who can be troublesome. Health institutions should clearly not move towards a style of management that totally disregards physicians as key employees with legitimate interests.

Physicians of the utmost fame
Were called at once; but when they came
They answered, as they took their fees,
'There is no cure for this disease.'

Hilaire Belloc

The Physician in Operations: Supplier and Marketer of Services

Physicians supply services and patients to an institution. They also use resources, thereby incurring costs to the institution. However, physicians are rarely salaried, full-time employees with related interests in the fiscal well-being of the institution. This, of course, is not the rule where organizations such as HMOs are concerned. This is also not true for group practices such as the South Clinic or Cleveland Clinic.

This section addresses two key issues brought about by the contradiction outlined above: first, fiscal and service relationships between health care institutions and independent groups of physicians which contract with institutions to provide selected services; and second, the physician as both marketer (revenue producer) and supplier of services (resource consumer).

Contracting with Physician Groups: The Case of Midland County Hospital

The general rule in the United States is that physicians practice on a fee-for-service basis and have affiliations at several hospitals. Increasingly however, physicians are forming groups that negotiate with the health organization. The power of such groups depends upon the alternatives which exist for the institution and the proportion of admissions produced by the physician group in its function as marketer. Even though such groups may appear to be independent entities whose internal workings are of no concern to the hospital chief executive officer, the fact is that once a contract is signed, the hospital becomes responsible for the activities of the group.

Midland County, like many community hospitals, has for years had its needs for radiological services provided by an arrangement with an independent group of radiologists. The hospital does not have any contract or any formal arrangements with this group. The group consists of two radiologists, one of whom chairs the Radiology Department. Both radiologists make their own arrangements with junior radiologists and with technicians.

Some years ago, there was an attempt to negotiate a contract but negotiations broke down. Because of what seemed to be an unusually high turnover rate within the group of radiologists, the administration of the hospital had become increasingly concerned about whether or not the group was, in fact, consistently able to staff the hospital's needs. This was a matter of concern not only to the administration. Fellow physicians were worried that the employees of the radiology group, despite their high qualifications, did not stay long within the hospital and that this turnover was partially attributable to the terms of employment opportunities offered by the group to its junior employees. From what the administration could gather, there were no formal contracts signed between the group and their employees, but the starting salary of $40,000 was generally increased by $4,000 at six-month intervals to a maximum of $60,000. Matters came to a head when three junior employees of the group approached the vice president for medical affairs and then the administrator of the hospital to complain about their employment situation. Each had somewhat different concerns: one had reached the maximum salary and wondered when he was going to get an increase, one was concerned with pregnancy benefits, and the third was concerned about what was going to happen to him given the treatment of the other two.

This dissatisfaction was of particular interest to the administration of Midland since they had just begun an attempt to negotiate an across-theboard contract with the radiology group, precipitated by a request from the group for an increase in their billing rates. The goal of the administration was to secure quality of care assurance from the group, as it was attempting to do with all groups in the hospital. The administration were concerned that this turnover, while primarily an internal matter for the group (and perhaps more broadly a matter for the medical executive committee of the hospital), was also indirectly a responsibility of the administration of the hospital, since it reflected upon the hospital's ability to guarantee quality of care.

As the contract negotiating process proceeded, the immediate concerns of two of the junior radiologists resolved themselves. One radiologist left for a more secure and better job elsewhere; the second went on an educational leave. The problem of the third junior radiologist remained unresolved.

The goal of the hospital on its side of the negotiations was to deal with the delicate matter of how the administration could secure its responsibilities without interfering directly with medical practice. To accomplish this, the administration attempted to place in the contract two provisions of particular note. One provision allowed the hospital administration to bring in outside experts to evaluate the department of radiology's performance. The second provision gave the hospital the right to review any change in the radiology group's membership that might actually or potentially affect the quality of care of the hospital. However, the central issue, turnover at existing staff levels, still had not been addressed in the draft of the contract provisions. The chief executive officer of the hospital wondered what he might put in the contract to provide some assurance that this persistent problem would diminish. He also wondered what other provisions should be in the contract that would give his administration some control over those aspects of the groups' functions that affected the hospital. However, he also wondered about resistance he might encounter from physicians objecting to these provisions as interference with medical practice.

A final complicating factor: the disaffected junior radiologist was actively pursuing the possibility of joining with two other radiologists, both of whom had worked successfully for the department in the past, to form a competing radiology group that would negotiate directly with the hospital. Since the radiology department at Midland is an open department, there was no reason why the administrator might not negotiate with this new group; but the CEO was apprehensive. Since the department head made the schedule for the department and was also the head of the other radiology group, he would obviously schedule his competition to look after all the Medicare and nonpaying cases. When the chief executive officer of Midland delicately approached the president of the medical staff to see how he thought the hospital's surgeons might react to the possibility of a second radiology group being formed, the president pointed out that the surgeons had been very happy with the existing group for many years, and it was unlikely that they would be enthusiastic about supporting a second group.

The Physician in Marketing and Production

The activities and behavior of the physician radically affect health care costs; institutional productivity; case mix; resource use, including the acquisition of technology; and quality of care. Since strategy is intimately concerned with these issues, decisions in these areas cannot be left to the discretion of physicians alone.

Productivity   The issue of productivity is important in two respects: first, there is much misinformation and misunderstanding about how productivity is measured and rewarded (if it is measured at all); second, there are informal expectations about productivity and service contributions which govern much of the behavior of physicians. With regard to the former, as health care organizations move from an implicit to an explicit strategy, there is greater need for more informed decisions on the part of both managers and physicians. This, in turn, implies better quality and sharing of information. If full involvement in significant decisions is to be obtained, then managers must keep their physicians informed.

At present, there is considerable subjectivity in most institutions. While a physician may wish to find out what revenue he or she produced for an institution in a given month, the information is not always readily available: "the numbers are too complicated to be explained to you." In fact, there is often a certain amount of necessary subjectivity built into the algorithm used to determine these data. For example, productivity standards are relative, not absolute; they vary by department, where they exist. Much in the way of improvement is desirable.

Promotion and Marketing   Marketing and promotional activities may be directed at attracting patients or attracting doctors. Such marketing programs share elements, whether they are directed to the immediate community, to potential patients outside that community, to referring physicians, or to physicians already on staff who may be potential purveyors of promotional programs. Promotional programs directed at attracting physicians should be sophisticated, mindful that, in addition to a specific job or career, the physician is interested in many aspects of the institution and community. Thus, information about and access to this whole spectrum may enhance the physician's interest. Physicians, however, should be recruited not simply on the basis of departmental need or desire but also on the basis of longer-range strategic considerations.

Hiring procedures should take the spouse and family into account. Amenities may range from the simple process of welcoming the spouse and ensuring the development of a network of friends and services, to helping the spouse find appropriate employment. Such measures have met with great success in the private sector, and there is reason to believe that they would be useful in the health sector.

Clarity is needed about the role of the board of trustees in hiring and the way in which physician salary and bonuses are computed. The financial aspects of hiring should not be secretive and should be open to negotiation. Some sort of management-by-objectives system, for example, might be instituted, whereby an agreement is made between the physician and the department concerning the former's role in revenue production. A physician's bonus might then be a function of his or her own willingness to work later or earlier or to develop a subspecialty. This should again take into account individual differences and variation in goals.

Doctor-Patient Mix   It is evident that each department of an institution, if left to its own devices, would quite naturally pursue strategic goals that are in its own interests. However, these goals might not always be in the best interests of the institution as a whole. Consequently, policy decisions should be made by the senior managers, both physician and non-physician, concerning growth directions for institutional departments. Moreover, these decisions should be reflected in *hiring* patterns. In fact, very different decisions might be made in the hiring of new physicians if managers were to ask three separate questions: If one could add one more patient visit, in which department should it take place? If one could add one more physician, in which department? And finally, if one could add one more patient, which geographic area, age group, or diagnostic group would you prefer that patient to represent? While these are obviously ideal questions, they underline the importance of using senior policymakers who can deal with the trade-offs inherent in these alternate strategic approaches.

These trade-offs become especially crucial as reimbursement systems begin to reward certain diagnostic-related group (DRG) mixes. In term of DRG-related payments at a clinic, a patient visit to an allergist or neurosurgeon may be preferable to one to acute medicine or dermatology, while in terms of adding another physician, an oral surgeon or a urologist may be more desirable than a pediatrician. Of course, not all patients will be suffering from undefined allergies or urological complications. Managerial trade-offs must be made among the different departments to utilize staff and facilities as effectively as possible. A further complication is that staffing must be adjusted to support growth or decrease of clinic visits in a certain department. It is critical for financial success that management be able to assess and dictate institutional growth patterns in such a way that, where necessary, trade-offs can be considered in terms of short- and long-run success.

Cost Management   It has been stated above that the latest reimbursement systems forces health delivery organizations to control costs but contain no direct incentives for physicians to do so. The situation at South Clinic is an intriguing example of the need to translate organizational cost-containment directives into physician incentive structures.

South Clinic consists of an out-patient clinic, run by a physician group practice, and a hospital to which these same physicians admit their patients for in-patient care. Different incentive systems exist in these interlocked but parallel institutions. In the hospital, the group practice physicians are paid on a fee-for-service basis. In other words, physicians receive their fee regardless of the costs they incur for the hospital. (The hospital's costs are similar to those of any other major teaching hospital's.) On the other hand, in the clinic, physicians are paid a salary plus bonus. Each physician has a set revenue target, i.e., he or she must generate enough patient revenues to cover the cost of his or her negotiated salary. Beyond that, each physician is paid a bonus out of a pool derived from the profits of the clinic. The profits are calculated as total revenues minus total costs. Each physician's bonus is allocated according to a formula based upon patient revenues plus other "weighted" contributions that the physician makes to the instituion. Since the level of the bonus is tied to the clinic's profit margin, physicians have an incentive to keep costs extremely low.

The Management of Technology   One problem that most health delivery organizations face is that physicians command organizational resources that concern direct service delivery, but they do not often have to manage capital or operating budgets. More and more hospitals are moving toward physician involvement in the latter budgets, but the penalty for doing so is that physicians can determine (or demand) the acquisition of technology which may or may not be affordable or reasonable. It is quite true that the costs of competition have become higher. Even the smallest hospital, whether planners like it or not, has to have a CAT scanner if it is to remain competitive. However, such technology can be acquired on a "for-use" basis and shared by institutions. There is an even more complex question about the use of technology in its generic sense; how is a health delivery institution to ensure that the latest and most effective technologies are brought into use promptly, while those that are ineffective are dropped? In the latter instance, there are potential resource issues. The National Institutes of Health, through the Office of Medical Applications of Research, has instituted consensus conferences which review new and outdated technology. But these conferences, while providing valuable information, have little, if any regulatory power. What is the manager of a hospital to do if he or she finds, for example, that surgeons are still practicing radical mastectomy for cases in which the consensus conference advises it not be used? While a multitude of review committees now exist in most hospitals, physicians on these committees are notoriously reluctant to dictate parameters for their peers' medical practices.

The Physician in Institutional Strategy

More and more physicians are recognizing the challenge of strategic management and are either receiving management training or becoming managers. However, the numbers are still too small to represent an adequate solution to the problem of how to involve the physician in strategic action when the competitive needs and interests of the organization as a whole diverge from those of the practicing clinician. For example, there has traditionally been competition between academic group practices and community physicians or groups. A dilemma faced by the formation of ambulatory care groups at teaching hospitals, such as those sponsored by the Robert Wood Johnson Foundation, is that these groups have to take care of a significant proportion of indigent patients and are thus marginally viable. As they seek to expand their market to become viable, they will inevitably come into competition with community physicians for non-indigent patients. This direction is resisted by the ambulatory group's own colleagues, subspecialists in the teaching hospital, who depend upon referral from the community physicians for their well-being. (They receive more referrals from the community than from their primary care colleagues.) There may be less of a conflict here in the future as the idea of separation diminishes and the possibility increases of teaching-hospital-based groups joining with community physicians in hybrid entities.

In conclusion, managers of today's health care institutions must give serious attention to the role of physicians in their institutions. Options for managing physician behavior and bringing it in line with the strategic objectives of the institution must take into account many factors, including size of the institution, type of governance, degree of physician domination, and history of the physician-institution relationship. A variety of approaches may be useful to administrators, including:

Physician education.

Use of more formal mechanisms for obtaining physician feedback (e.g., the use of a survey by HCAN).

Direct financial incentives.

Alternative investment opportunities.

Peer support and feedback groups.

Use of high-status role models to encourage behavior/attitudinal modification.

These approaches fall into one of two categories. The first is rationale; the second is power. Managers must ask, in the first case, to what extent physicians are informed about and understand the relationship between what they do and the consequences of what they do, such as outcome and costs for the patient and for society. Are they aware of variations and the situational factors that cause variations? Are standards clear, known, and rational? Are standards communicated? Do standards become expectations?

With regard to power, do managers rely on advocates or pressure groups representing more or less desirable behaviors? How are physicians selected for employment, and what values do they manifest in relation to institutional goals? Are there graded sanctions or rewards for physician compliance? For the most part, the tendency is first to educate or bring to bear group pressure on physicians and then to shift sharply to more extreme measures, such as denying hospital affiliation or payment. Be aware, however, that no system can operate effectively if it vacillates between vague, minor pressures and extreme, absolute, or inappropriate pressures. A graded system is required.

The answer lies in the creation of incentive systems that make desirable to physicians the behavior which a health institution requires, rather than in attempting to control divergent behavior. Such incentive systems are only now beginning to be considered. Clearly there are two major elements: (1) management's desire for certain behaviors from physicians must be clearly understood and specified; (2) the incentives must be responsive to the motivations of the physician. Money is a powerful motivator, but it is not everything. Physicians also want a reasonable life and the opportunity to practice what they consider to be good medicine.

Summary

Physician and institutional interests, once synonymous, have diverged. Doctors attempt to preserve traditional autonomies in practice patterns, while hospitals seek to curb costs and respond to communities. As institutions become concerned with productivity, case mix, and costs, past mechanisms for managing physicians no longer work. The physician's role as occasional participant is threatened when the organization of which he or she is a member moves in unfamiliar and possibly uncomfortable directions. Doctors, if they are not to become totally alienated, must become more involved in institutional strategy and performance. This involvement will take the form of new types of governance and innovative incentive schemes.

Issues in Competitive Strategy

CHAPTER

8

Chiefly the mould of a man's fortune is in his own hands.

Francis Bacon

This chapter starts with a long case example—as a summary of many of the issues raised in the previous chapters—and goes on to recap the strategic alternatives. Then the major types of health organizations are briefly discussed, and some of the strategic issues associated with each. Finally, some general strategic issues are raised.

A Case Example: South Clinic

Identifying an organization's existing competitive strategy, position, and performance is key, since these must first be understood if they are to be evaluated and changed. Since many health organizations have implicit (i.e., unstated and unarticulated) strategies and few unequivocal measures for evaluating performance, this identification is not always as easy as it might seem. South Clinic is an example in point.

South Clinic is a medical group practice organized as a partnership of physicians with 85 partners; it is run by a board of management of 7 doctors. The administration includes a medical director, associate and assistant medical directors, and a sizable administrative staff. The clinic employs many doctors in addition to the partners, and has a total of 650 employees. The partnership rents the clinic building from the South Medical Foundation, and its partners use the Foundation Hospital. A non-profit corporation, South Medical Foundation has several operating divisions; major ones include the Foundation Hospital (1,869 employees), the graduate medical education division, the school of allied health sciences, and the research institute. The president of the foundation is also chief executive officer of the hospital (a recent innovation) and there is a board of trustees of 51 members and an executive committee of 15 members, 7 of whom are physicians; each of the latter is also a partner in the clinic. The foundation has 107 employees working outside the hospital in such additional foundation divisions as finance, employee relations, planning and development, and public affairs. There is also a service corporation whose stock is held solely by people who work at the medical institutions; this corporation owns and operates a hotel and affiliated services.

The president, newly appointed, felt that it was time to reconsider South Clinic's strategy in the light of recent developments.

If one attempts to articulate South Clinic's strategy in the light of a rigorous definition of the term, much is lacking. Indeed, the clinic's only explicit strategy has been the rather vague formulation, "to achieve the highest level of patient care in a setting of medical education and medical investigation." Clearly, something more is required if this organization is to deal with the complexities presented by an increasingly regulated and competitive environment. Not only must a clear and unambiguous strategy be defined, but appropriate steps must be taken to see that it becomes a reality. So South Clinic began a definitional process.

Inasmuch as the South Clinic institutions had no explicit strategy or clear-cut measures of performance, a variety of activities were started in an attempt to define the implicit strategy as clearly as possible and then to assess its viability. To do this, the patient population was analyzed and significant trends in its mix and volume were identified to help pinpoint any particular problems or opportunities. A separate but connected look at financial status was made. Information for both of these studies came from existing clinical and financial data. One important difficulty arose, however; data often did not exist or were difficult to obtain. This was generally due to the nature of the existing information systems, which were incomplete or incompatible.

The second step was to examine the question of physician recruitment and retention. This was an important part of the study, since decisions about patient mix and procedures result, in large part, from prior decisions about the kinds of physicians recruited and retained. As such, these decisions are critical to determining the existing and future well-being of any medical institution. To do this, a number of physicians were interviewed, some of whom had considered coming to South Clinic and had subsequently decided to go elsewhere, and others who had accepted positions at the clinic.

The third step was to analyze the ways in which South Clinic attracted patients, i.e., its promotional strategies. Much of this work had already been carried out in a prior public relations study, which was now augmented. The final step was to analyze the present and future environment in which South Clinic operated. Interviews with senior decision makers led to the conclusion that the clinic essentially defined itself as a major regional resource rather than as a national health care institution. This definition led to an understanding of what South Clinic's strategy had been.

South Clinic is a large medical group practice which implies a desire to share in the control of patient care activities and to have those patient care activities be of a general rather than a highly specialized nature. The provision of clinical care, in fact, is more important than research or education, and is addressed to the region rather than to the immediate locality or the nation. Doctors in the partnership desire a good rather than an extraordinary income, and an average rather than an excessive volume of work. This unemphatic style has been carried over into the way in which the institution presents itself to the public.

Its implicit strategy has been to offer a broad range of high-quality patient care to a wide spectrum of patients from a local and regional area, with a smattering of international patients. There has been no particular concentration of activities in terms of either specialties or type of patient. The strategy has not been implemented aggressively, as there have been few promotional activities geared to either patients or physicians. As a result, growth has occurred at a rate somewhat less than the growth rate of the market served. A further consequence of South Clinic's unaggressive promotional effort has been that the competitive actions of other institutions have led to shifts in the clinic's patient mix toward primary care and away from subspecialty care, as well as to an apparent increase in the number of patients entering through the emergency room. This is not the result of deliberate action on the part of the South Clinic institutions; rather, it is strategy by inaction or default. A reflection of the clinic's identity, and an aspect of its undefined and unaggressive promotional efforts, is that the physicians are generally less productive than they were four years ago. Although the lowered productivity may be explained by the increased attention to research and teaching on the part of some physicians, an explicit strategy which would dictate such a shift is lacking. Further, a shift to cost-based Medicaid and Medicare payment, with collection difficulties, has resulted in lags in reimbursement and, correspondingly, an increase in accounts receivable.

The major trends identified in the environment are that the market is likely to continue to grow, at least in the short term, especially in the adult and elderly populations and in the number of women of childbearing age. However, the very rapid growth of local and regional competing institutions which are strengthening existing programs and developing new ones can be expected to cut sharply into South Clinic's share of the market.

Competitively, then, South Clinic's strategy (implicit) has been low-growth, on-site, and somewhat differentiated—but essentially maintenance in nature. Until now, success for South has come from a favorable competitive position rather than from effective implementation of explicit strategy. Implicitly, also, the clinic has engaged in a "differentiated" strategy. It is the only group practice providing a full range of quality care in a competitive market consisting of community and teaching hospitals, and is therefore able to attract high-quality physicians. As this strategy is projected forward, the following conclusions appear.

Consequences of Strategy Continuation without Change: The Likely Scenario

The point of a group practice is twofold: first, the group should have a greater degree of control over its medical fate than would individuals in solo practice or in an organization under the control of others. Secondly, group members may refer patients to one another and, therefore, have the collective satisfaction of dealing with a wide range of patients over a long span of time. Ideally, perhaps, a group practice would like to offer lifetime care to some portion of its patients. Given the absence of competition, this goal might well be largely achievable, although subject to the vagaries of population shifts. This goal further ensures that doctors who find each other compatible, and whose specialties are complementary, are able to provide care for a varied group of patients with a great deal of professional satisfaction. In addition, such activities ensure an income level which provides both for the continuation of the organization and the maintenance of a preferred lifestyle for physicians.

What has happened to South Clinic is that there have been small but increasingly rapid shifts in patients' ability to pay, in reimbursement mechanisms, and in competitive actions by other institutions. The market of "captive" patients who might use the clinic as their lifetime medical resource and who are able to pay for such care, either directly or through insurance, has decreased. The result is a diminishing supply of patients for subspecialists and a consequent replacement of internal referrals by other sources of patients and income. These new arrangements have included relationships of various kinds with other institutions, in the hope that referrals would occur. Additionally, the international market has been approached somewhat more aggressively than in the past. But activities directed towards increasing primary care referrals, through affiliation with other institutions or by increasing primary care services within South Clinic itself, are relatively inefficient; the lack of an intrinsic relationship between physician and patient means that many patients may seek their secondary or tertiary care elsewhere. Indeed, the dilemma is exacerbated when, as has been the case, young physicians who have learned a particularly "caring" approach at South Clinic move elsewhere. Ironically, there are many such physicians who today represent a significant source of competition for the clinic.

As other institutions continue to develop excellent primary care units as well as highly competent tertiary referral units, South Clinic's monopoly over its group of "lifetime" patients is likely to diminish further. Moreover, the clinic's capacity to differentiate itself competitively from the community hospitals (e.g., by attracting excellent physicians) is diminishing. To ensure a sufficient number of subspecialty referrals, South Clinic will have to emphasize even more primary care, either at the main campus or by establishing satellites. This will mean a heavier workload for physicians because of the additional patient load and the consequent emphasis on increased productivity. The shift to more general care will, in turn, make the institution less attractive to the ambitious and excellent physician, thereby further diminishing the clinic's ability to attract the best doctors.

The ultimate consequence for South Clinic of continuing its present strategy is twofold: a leveling out of care, and a different, probably lower-quality, physician staff (both the result of increased demand on and lower income for the physician). Since the linkage between the clinic and hospital is so strong, both organizations can be expected to suffer if one suffers.

It is possible that this scenario would be acceptable to the partnership, but it is unlikely. There is a need for an explicit statement of identity and goals, coupled with an agreement concerning the tasks necessary to achieve such an identity. Indeed, in light of the environment and the distinctive competence of the institutions, some new directions seem called for. In making this assertion, there are three key assumptions:

South Clinic wishes to remain a group practice with a compatible and excellent group of doctors.

These doctors want to have a varied and interesting mix of care activities for a varied and interesting group of patients.

The institution wishes to be able to support these activities and maintain a good but not excessive income for the physicians.

Based on these assumptions, the specific strengths and weaknesses of South Clinic may be detailed.

Essential strengths are:

A staff dedicated to patient care and well trained in multiple specialties.

An image as a first-rate institution.

A history and tradition in its local area as an innovator and trend setter.

A superb physical plant where space still exists for growth and where hotel facilities exist for foreign patients.

Teaching affiliations which bring through a number of young physicians who are likely to be sources for referral and/or future membership in the partnership.

A cadre of good managers and a smaller group of physicians who are prepared to take on additional responsibilities outside the main institution, and who have done so in the past.

Weaknesses include:

A lack of organizational definition, identity, and strategy, resulting in inadvertent consequences. This weakness, in fact, prompted the study.

Ambiguous information sharing within the institution that has led to some dissention and conflict. Conflict also exists with elements outside the institution, resulting in occasionally incorrect perceptions of many aspects of South Clinic's function.

Decisions about hiring that have not taken a broader strategy into account.

Lack of sufficient connection between the clinic and the hospital. This has led to numerous problems, including difficulties in tracing information and charges and variability in physician time. Lack of a well-integrated relationship between clinic and hospital has also resulted in a loss of the flexibility and activity coordination that often come from a more consolidated operation.

Strategy and Values

A fairly explicit aspect of South Clinic's strategy is the relatively small emphasis placed on research. This is reflected both in the amount of funding available for research and in a pervasive attitude among physicians which discourages interest in activities that are not directly related to patient care. Education is highly valued, but most of the activities are directed—with the exception of training residents—toward nonphysician training. In fact, while many doctors may have medical school appointments, few appear to spend much time in that form of education. Ongoing research appears to be divided between basic research on a small number of topics and a certain amount of applied clinical research. Although it seems clear that this lack of emphasis on research is an explicit choice, it is not clear that the implication of such a choice for tertiary care referrals has been as fully considered as it might be. Indeed, this choice has already had consequences in terms of the kinds of physicians attracted to South Clinic, and it may have further consequences for physician turnover.

Certain of the available strategic choices involve a somewhat different emphasis on research or education. It should be pointed out that any shift in emphasis is not just a matter of allocating resources, such as money or space, but in changing attitudes which make time spent on these activities relatively unacceptable to the present group of physicians. The impetus behind this reviewing strategy was a concern about certain past trends and their implications for the future. South Clinic's implicit strategy to date has begun to have dysfunctional effects on the identity of the institutions. Significant changes, however, seem to be unnecessary to regain control over key aspects of the clinic's identity and to assure the institutions' viability in an increasingly complex, competitive, and regulated environment.

Essentially, what is uncovered here is a set of values about certain kinds of patients, doctors, and patient care activities, and certain work, income, and career conditions. The major physician values appear to revolve around patient care and an appropriate sharing of such care. It is possible to operationalize some of these dimensions, i.e., create objectives by asking for views about desirable diagnosis and patient origins, subspecialties, kinds of physician, and levels of income and productivity.

These values have considerable implications and consequences as constraints upon new directions. For example, it would obviously be necessary to put greater resources into research if that is to be emphasized, either as a way of attracting physicians or as a route to developing new technologies that will give South Clinic a distinctive competence and, thus, an edge in the market. But this investment alone is insufficient; to be effective it requires a concomitant attitude change toward greater tolerance of nonclinical activities stemming from different measurements of productivity and different dissemination of such measures. There appears to be little understanding on the part of highly productive clinicians that dissemination of research findings can be an extraordinarily effective promotional tool bringing in considerable revenue.

Possible Products

A useful way to think about the set of elements involving kinds of patients, subspecialists, or primary care purveyors, is to consider that South Clinic essentially offers *at least* four "products:"

1. Lifelong Care This is offered to a "captive" group of patients and provides them with all necessary care, primary through tertiary, at all stages of life. Group practices are particularly suited to providing such a service, although prepaid group practices have achieved an edge here.

2. Primary Care While a proportion has always been offered by South Clinic, this has been increasing. This may be a relatively inefficient way of providing referrals to subspecialties and may require a higher volume than captive, lifelong patients.

3. Diagnostic Workups For people in good health, the provision of routine physicals, i.e., diagnostic workups, has become a very lucrative source of revenue for many health institutions. (This is a highly competitive field.) Diagnostics for sick patients is also an increasing source of revenue, especially in the international market South Clinic seeks.

4. Major Therapeutic Procedures Especially those which result in hospital admission for the above categories of patient. However, there are few direct admissions to the South Hospital without attendance at the clinic first. This is presumably because of the intrinsic link between clinic and hospital: the clinic drives the hospital. The consequence, however, is that hospital beds can go unfilled when the clinic's volume diminishes or its case mix changes toward more primary care. Unfortunately, occupancy problems cannot be solved by direct action of the hospital.

It will be important for South Clinic to consider the above products, along with any others which might be identified, in conjunction with the key elements of the institutions' identity and distinctive competence. Such consideration should accompany a review of the strategic alternatives below.

The Strategic Alternatives: What Do They Look Like?

1. Low Growth: Maintenance and/or Differentiation In this strategy, the goal of South Clinic is to maintain everything which it now does and values, but at a level of activity that will not result in losses due to competitive erosion or inflation. This inevitably means that there must be, in fact, some growth in the volume of activities and the income derived therefrom.

In the next two strategy options, the goal is to retain the same set of basic activities but at an enhanced level.

2. Onsite High Growth: Maintenance and/or Differentiation The major growth occurs on the main campus. This involves increased effort and an emphasis on promotional and referral activities. It must obviously be specified whether the growth is primarily in income, volume, or kind of activities. Efforts should be made to sharpen the distinctive image of South Clinic.

3. Offsite High Growth: Maintenance and/or Differentiation   The major growth occurs in satellites away from the main campus and involves a number of options. Satellite development can occur through acquisition, merger, affiliation, or management or clinical contracts. Essentially, the goal is to increase revenues and patients without enlarging the staff on the main campus. Again, a distinctive image is crucial.

The following strategies involve major shifts in basic activities.

4. Focus   Fewer activities than previously, and the institutions become more highly specialized. This may involve emphasizing research and/or education, becoming more of a national referral center, or developing expertise in a small number of subspecialties. The assumption is that by allocating large amounts of resources to certain specified areas, South Clinic can obtain a market edge in these areas.

5/6. Diversification/Mini-Health-System   The shift here is into a wider range of activities. The goal is to secure stability and growth by engaging in more and different kinds of patient-care activities, or by establishing more and different sources of revenue. Patient-care alternatives might include the acquisition of health institutions or the creation of innovative forms of care such as surgicenters. Alternative sources of revenue might include extensions of existing activity, such as management contracts or even the purchase of non-health care, income-producing ventures. These alternative revenue sources would allow the central institution to continue providing service for which it is at least partially subsidized.

Any of these options are theoretically possible, but options 2 and 3 require considerable investment and, given the rapid increase in size, would effect the greatest overall change. Option 4 is probably unpalatable to South Clinic, though Cleveland Clinic's strategy (discussed earlier) has been to invest heavily in research as a way of getting a competitive edge in new technology. Options 5/6 are also unlikely to be aggressively pursued, as they had been tried by a previous (lay) president who wound up too far ahead of the physicians and out of a job. The strategy likely to fit best with values and resources, therefore, is option 1, or a modest version of option 2 or 3. But *differentiation* is critical to keeping a favorable competitive position and performance. Without differentiation, maintenance would likely result in further erosion of South Clinic's position.

Whether differentiation is indeed possible, or whether a distinctive image can be reestablished and effectively communicated—these questions must be faced squarely before any strategy is adopted. If not, then South Clinic will increasingly be seen as just another goodish hospital.

Nothing more certain than uncertainties
Fortune is full of fresh variety
Constant in nothing but inconstancy.

Richard Barnfield

Sectors of the Industry

Teaching Hospitals   These have always been the flagships of the industry. They have led the way in research and provided the exemplar to the new generations of professionals. In some instances, they have led the way in managerial innovation: Johns Hopkins was one of the first, if not the very first, to develop a responsibility-based, departmental budgeting system. But with cost consciousness rising, the problem of paying for teaching has become paramount. As community hospitals have grown and become wealthy enough to steal away the excellent physicians, the best medical practice is being spread around. With the advent of diagnosis-related groups, teaching hospitals have to enrich their patient mixes if they are to be reimbursed at an adequate level. The Robert Wood Johnson Foundation has taken the lead in helping transform relatively conservative medical departments into vital group practices. But the problems remain. How can teaching hospitals, often located in difficult urban areas, provide care to the indigent and also pay for their excellence? One critical problem lies in the fear of competition with the community physicians who refer to the teaching hospitals much of the subspecialty case load. If a teaching hospital aggressively pursues paying patients, community physicians will be up in arms. And since many, if not most, of the physicians in a teaching hospital are salaried faculty, there is a critical problem in motivation. As the emphasis moves from excellence in research and teaching to productivity, will academic medical centers develop the necessary incentive mechanisms to reward the physician behavior necessary to their survival?

As supergroups and alliances (see below) begin to dominate the industry and aggregate resources, will the traditional teaching hospital continue to flourish as it has? Teaching hospitals cannot simply join them if they can't fight them. If these academic centers become too enmeshed in productive clinical practice, their major role will be blurred. And finally, but by no means least, if the physician glut that is promised comes about, and teaching hospitals have to cut back on their central function, how will they maintain even this role? New England Medical Center is experimenting with becoming the low-cost, high-quality supplier to HMOs. But even as it moves in this direction, Health Maintenance Organizations are becoming concerned about the high cost of referring patients to excessively expensive teaching institutions. The HMO's response is to acquire their own institutions or to use excellent community hospitals with lower costs. One possible counterresponse for teaching hospitals is to develop academic group practices. But, although these provide income for academic physicians, they do little to alter the motivational incentive systems. And they do bring academic faculty into direct conflict with community doctors.

Teaching hospitals with a strong base in technology will probably continue to have an edge as long as they attend to disseminating their innovations. But it is not too farfetched to expect a development similar to that in Great Britain, where there has been a significant reduction in the number of teaching hospitals.

Community Hospitals   These face a different set of issues, With a far greater variety of size and capability, they cannot really be evaluated as a single entity. Smaller community hospitals in noncompetitive situations may well be able to continue to flourish. However, any community hospital under 250 beds in a competitive situation is doomed to failure unless it merges with some larger entity. And even the larger community hospitals are finding comfort in collaboration. Lacking the constraints facing the teaching hospitals, which fear collaboration because of dilution of quality, most community hospitals of any size are aggressively seeking merger or association with larger groupings. The cost of competition is entirely too great for the independent, autonomous institution to endure.

The strategies of community hospitals are marked by two major developments—association into ever larger groupings and specialization into sophisticated market segments. St. Mary's Hospital, a small, 200-bed community hospital in Newark, seeks to enlarge its Roman Catholic network. St. James Hospital, a simiiarly sized Catholic institution, takes a different route. It seeks to dominate the local area by capturing primary care referral sources, and it has carved out a fascinating market by providing occupational health programs to surrounding commercial establishments. Through association with a larger alliance, Dale Medical Center seeks to be able to provide its smaller hospital brethren in the locality with management services. The smaller hospitals that do not merge generally join some kind of alliance or association that will provide a higher quality of management services than they could otherwise afford. Recognizing the need for referral and disposal, community hospitals integrate vertically, if large enough on their own, or through the medium of a hospital group. And, while individual practice is still a strongly held value in many parts of the country, and fee for service is still a banner under which many march, even the smallest community hospital is beginning to salary its department chairperson.

Group Practice   New forms of group practice are beginning to appear everywhere. Whether in a single specialty or multispecialty arrangement, physicians recognize that by combining they can control more than is possible individually. Many smaller group practices still are essentially for physicians only. But it is only a matter of time before physicians recognize that owning their support staff and equipment will enable them to generate retainable revenues. The larger group practices seem to be flourishing. They have led the way in incentive innovations that will filter down to other types of institutions. And their combination of management and medical expertise, with physicians in the driver's seat, represents one strategic direction for the future.

Independent Practice Associations (IPAs)   These developed originally as a response to **Health Maintenance Organizations (HMOs)**. Both recognized the advantage of the prepaid system as a way of controlling health care costs. Straddling three businesses—insurance, prevention, and care—they face the delicate issue of managing the healthy/sick ratio. The only way you make money in the prepaid business is by keeping sick costs low and the healthy/sick ratio high. Many HMOs are finding that if they are too good at providing sick care, healthy patients are lost and costs rise. Keeping sick costs down involves using relatively low-cost hospitals that are geographically proximate. The problem of combining insurance and health care mechanisms is that the insurance mechanism is independent of distance, while people needing care want to get it close by. Where do you refer? Do you build a new hospital or a condominium wing on an existing one? How does an IPA, which reimburses the member physician on a fee-for-service basis, control that physician's pattern of practice? How can an HMO, which can only expand by building a new center, expand as easily and successfully as an IPA? And how can both live up to the promises of prevention which have yet to be realized?

Hospital Groups   Such groups of various forms have become the fashionable entity in health care. But like their larger brethren, the alliances and supergroups, they have to date promised more than they have performed. Relatively few true mergers have yet occurred, in the sense of full integration and reallocation of resources. Nor is it at all evident that such entities reduce costs. They are, however, highly competitive in that they provide greater resources and more opportunities for diversified services. Like their larger brethren, they remain brittle, an uncomfortable combination of collaboration and competition. The advent of the Preferred Provider Option (PPO) may provide the cement, in the form of incentives. Geographically based hospital groups have the potential for providing a fully integrated range of services to a catchment area. But many are finding that it is easier to engage principally in the peripheral services that require less integration and may be more attractive financially. Such would include management contracting and shared services.

Super Groups   Over the past six years, groups of groups, or so-called super groups, have emerged; and for the first time it seems at least possible that the "cottage industry" will become truly "industrial." Such innovations are appearing mostly in the western states. Health Network has $653 million in assets and owns or manages 18 hospitals. It will engage in new developments, resource allocation, planning, marketing, and financial planning. Its goals are to get economies of scale, to develop shared services, and to encourage vertical integration and experimentation. It hopes to compete on price for regional and national PPOs. The Adventist Health System had over 100 hospitals in 1980, with 9,300 beds and assets of more than $1 billion. Health Frontiers, in the same year, had many smaller hospitals with assets over $150 million; its goal is to provide a regional network while retaining local ownership. The Voluntary Hospital Association, starting from a base of cooperative buying and consciously providing an alternative to the investor-owned systems, is well on its way to its five-year goal of 100 hospitals, 60,000 beds, and $8 billion in revenues. Recently, it bought 25 percent of a financial services company (in which the Mellon Bank has a minority interest). It plans to provide its members with a range of services by helping them develop first the feasibility studies and then the resources themselves, including retirement centers, primary care centers, emergicenters, surgicenters, alcohol units, and other add-ons. It will also stimulate management contracting, especially through a subsidiary, the Health Ventures Company, which will develop HMOs, IPAs, and PPOs. Such massive endeavors are beginning to provoke antitrust issues.

Alliances   Paralleling these super groups are the alliances. The Associated Hospitals System (AHS), a joint venture company, has 150 hospitals, with 30,000 beds, 250 management contracts, and over $1.8 billion in revenues. This loosely held organization will share information and software and will eventually add strategic planning and shared services. It plans cooperative ventures, pooling of resources, and counseling on specific issues. Membership fees for some of these large organizations range from $30,000 for each multi-hospital system that joins AHS, to $75,000 for a share in the Voluntary Hospital Association. Is the membership fee worth it? Evidently a lot of hospitals think so.

Strategically, the supergroups and alliances are competing with the for-profits. As cuts in Medicare and Medicaid occur, these groups want to maximize reimbursement for their members from other sources. Their massive size means that they have an edge in competing for capital. They can provide shared services and strategic planning in a way that the smaller groups, let alone individual institutions, cannot manage. They are in a marvellous position to offer PPO options to national employers on a highly competitive basis. One key strategic difference between super-groups and alliances is that while alliances are essentially joint ventures for specific purposes, with no control over members, supergroups like Health Network do have broad power over members with committed assets. The strategic issue yet to be fully faced is exactly what these large groupings constitute. Are they large support entities intended to help the individual institution compete successfully in its own area and provide excellent health care, or are they national companies offering health care on a regional or national basis? And can health care be provided in that way?

Health Centers   What are the strategic problems of the smaller entities? Health centers, developed under federal funding, are now drying up. A social innovation created under essentially social welfare legislation, such centers have provided badly needed health care in urban and rural areas. Can and should they survive? The Neponset Health Center in Boston is attempting to redirect its activities toward paying patients. But if it is successful, will it still serve its original social function? There is a tendency in health care to assume that any organizational innovation, once it exists, has a right to continue. Can health centers such as Neponset successfully shift their strategic efforts? Should they? And if they do not, who will pick up the slack? At this point, there is a delicate conflict between social policy and institutional strategy

Nursing Homes   One of the major issues facing most Western societies in the next two decades is the growing burden of the very old, very sick. This will affect not only the nursing home industry but also the hospital industry. The average age of the occupants of many nursing homes is well over 75 years. And as the progress of technology keeps ever more sick, old people alive, nursing homes will have to deal with more complex patients. This issue has barely been confronted. Does the answer lie in developing *nursing home groups* that will offer, as Nursing Homes Associated does, both protected living arrangements and sophisticated nursing homes, or in the integration of extended care with acute care systems? Should the very old be institutionalized or kept at home?

Home Health Agencies   The fringe of this issue spills over into the strategic dilemmas of the home health agencies. The Visiting Nurse Association of Denver, as described above, now faces competition from some 22 other agencies, and this situation is repeated in many other cities. Can a single home health agency deal with the full range of problems it faces, or should it specialize and develop new entities? How can the highly specialized resources required to keep the aged independent and able be best organized and brought to bear on the problem?

For-Profits   Behind many of the competitive concerns raised above lies the specter of the for-profits. Their competitive edge has lain until now in the excellence of their management. But developments in the past half decade have shown that the voluntary sector can match the for-profits in management excellence. Despite reservations that may not always be untrue, the for-profit sector has demonstrated that good management can pay off in health care. But will the voluntary institutions end up making the same mistakes and having the same accusations leveled at them as the for-profits have? It is disturbing to talk to the head of a voluntary hospital group and hear him describe physicians as his potential competitors.

Some General Strategic Issues

Competition in the health field has, until recently, revolved around patients and doctors. How can you get the best possible care to those who need it? In the recent past, competition has centered on management issues. How can you get the best possible management to the organizations that need it or that do not yet have it? How can you manage institutions so that they may make money here to pay for care there? But the emerging issue—which is economic, moral, medical, and strategic—is the fact that as technology makes it possible to keep ever more people alive, the cost of doing so can no longer be afforded. Not every child with a failing liver can be kept alive. Not every baby with brain damage can be restored to full capacity. Not every 80-year-old with a third stroke can be rehabilitated. And while this is basically a social issue, it does become a strategic issue for the individual institution. How is the institution going to allocate its resources to those in most need?

If competition in the past has focused on patients, doctors, and managers, a critical issue now is *strategic training*. Looking forward, General Electric recognized that it needed to develop in high school students an interest in engineering. In the health field, there is a need to develop people now who will have the skills, abilities, and attitudes required by the health system of the future. There is a need for a new breed of professionals/managers, nurses, doctors, and technicians, who will be able to combine professional (and humane) skills with managerial abilities. This is more than simply deciding whether there is a need for more or fewer physicians or nurses in the next decade. It is more than deciding for the umpteenth time whether one should increase or decrease the capacity of a medical school or should shut down nondegree nursing schools. It involves new kinds of training, both for existing professionals, as well as for new and different kinds of professionals. As the health field moves from a cottage industry to big business, it has to recognize that strategic training is a crucial issue, and that such training requires much lead time if it is to be integrated into curricula.

At a more prosaic level, it is important to recognize that *strategic change* needs attention. Traditionally, there has been relatively little "management slack" in the health industry. Or "professional slack" for that matter. Everybody is very busy with what they normally do. Yet the changes described in this book are so pervasive and so profound that specific attention must be paid to them. This requires time and effort. Hospitals merge, and yet their chief executive officers go on doing what they did before. Group practices are formed, yet the physicians in charge of them go on doing their research and clinical practice as though their managerial responsibilities were minor. There is no orderly progression, but the helter-skelter flight of the lemmings. Jobs must be redefined and time for reflection must be built in, if the "caring" industry is truly to care.

These changes—economic, political, social, ethical, technological, educational, medical—are indeed profound. The world in which patients and health care professionals have lived is altering radically. It is a paradigm change. It may not even be possible to get from here to there without the careful design of transitional organizations in which the purpose is to alter attitudes and values that will only result in changed behavior farther down the road. If organizations are to share resources, their members need to learn how not to own. Given the weight of history, it is probably not surprising that even in wholly owned hospital groups, individual top managers still behave as though they were working for individual hospitals. What is more surprising is the lack of attention and time paid to this issue.

The health field has traditionally been hierarchical. Doctors, boards, and top managers have run things. Yet there are many superb ideas that come from staff members when they are given an opportunity. One key strategic issue for the health industry, as it moves toward ever larger aggregation, is how to combine big business with a participative management based upon practical politics. Those that deal with the patients and the issues are often ahead of those that deal with the philosophies and strategies. Can health organizations conjure up the trick of being big and bold and small and beautiful at the same time?

Postscript

This book has dealt with the pragmatic aspects of competitive strategy. If you run some kind of health institution, what can you do to be successful? The book has not attempted to deal with the personal, moral, or ethical issues involved. There are larger social issues, as alluded to in the last section. Social policy, ultimately, has to determine how resources are allocated and to whom.

Will competition in the health field provide better quality of care to those who need it? The answer can only be equivocal. To the extent that competition centers on cost, quality probably will not be hurt badly, and competition over quality will have to result in at least slight and technical improvements. It is my personal view that freedom lies in having alternatives. If competition encourages the health care system to give people alternatives, to that extent the quality of lives may be improved. Will a young woman be able to choose between a radical mastectomy and a lumpectomy with radiation? Will a sick old man be free to choose between a nursing home and care in his own home? Will the patient have access to a system that understands and gives meaning to people's lives? The answer can only be equivocal.

What about those who have rarely had health care, except at the indulgence of the system? There has been a long and great tradition of institutions and physicians giving charity care, i.e., care that comes out of their hides. This became a right in more recent years with the advent of Medicare and Medicaid, though there are still many who do not qualify and who are still treated as a personal or organizational responsibility. Every time we legislate a right, it costs someone. Perhaps as we develop the Preferred Provider Option (PPO), giving industry the opportunity to cut its benefit costs significantly through discounts which will help institutions and professionals make a profit, we should add an override. If all PPO options had a 5(?) percent override put into a fund for those who could not afford care, the private sector could make a major contribution to those whom the federal government seems increasingly reluctant to help.

What about the overproduction of physicians? The general conclusion seems to be that this may do little to reduce health care costs and a lot to help competition. Perhaps we should borrow a solution from the agricultural sector, where farmers producing corn that is not needed are paid not to produce, and put our excess physicians out to pasture. Since physicians are believed to generate a major proportion of the costs of health care, we might save large sums by paying them not to practice.

And what about the supergroups? As managerial dominance replaces physician dominance, will we see a rebellion of doctors? As major companies sew up the jobs, will we witness a strange phenomenon: physicians forming unions, becoming a moral labor force standing for what is right and humane against the bottom-line arguments of management?

It all comes down to one thing. For all the marvels of management and technology, you and I, too, are eventually going to get sick and we are going to die. And before that, we will have small things go wrong with us. Will *we* find someone in this health care system who understands us and can help us in the way we want to be helped, who understands the meaning of *our* lives? That is the problem and the blessing of working in health care; our lives are entwined with it as professionals and as future patients. Whether competitive strategy ultimately works for the well-being of people as well as for the well-being of organizations, depends on what we *all* find when we need help ourselves.

General References

Abell, Derek F. *Defining the Business: The Starting Point of Strategic Planning.* Englewood Cliffs, N.J.: Prentice-Hall, 1980.

Aldrich, Howard, E. *Organizations and Environments.* Englewood Cliffs, N.J.: Prentice-Hall, 1979.

Barrett, Diana. *Multihospital Systems: The Process of Development.* Cambridge, Mass.: Oelgeschlager, Gunn and Hain, 1980.

Berger, John, and Mohr, Jean. *A Fortunate Man.* New York: Pantheon Books, 1967.

Bower, Joseph L. *Managing the Resource Allocation Process: Study of Corporate Planning and Investment.* Boston: Harvard University Division of Research, Graduate School of Business Administration, 1970.

Chandler, Alfred D., Jr. *Strategy and Structure.* Cambridge: Massachusetts Institute of Technology, 1962.

_____. *The Visible Hand: The Managerial Revolution in American Business.* Cambridge, Mass.: The Belknap Press, 1977.

Cooper, Philip D., ed. *Health Care Marketing.* Germantown, Md.: Aspen Systems, 1979.

Drucker, Peter F. *Management, Tasks, Responsibilities, Practices.* New York: Harper & Row, 1973.

Emery, F. E., and Trist, E. L. *Toward a Social Ecology: Contextual Appreciation of the Future in the Present.* London: Plenum Press, 1973.

Goldsmith, J. C. *Can Hospitals Survive? The New Competitive Health Care Market.* Homewood, Ill.: Dow Jones-Irwin, 1981.

Hirschman, Albert O. *Shifting Involvements: Private Interest and Public Action.* Princeton, N.J.: Princeton University Press, 1982.

Jaques, Elliott, ed. *Health Services: Their Nature and Organization and the Role of Patients, Doctors, and the Health Professions.* London: Heinemann Educational Books, 1978.

Kimberly, John R., Robert H. Miles and Associates. *The Organizational Life Cycle.* San Francisco: Jossey-Bass, 1980.

Kotler, Philip. *Marketing Management Analysis, Planning and Control.* 4th ed. Englewood Cliffs, N.J.: Prentice-Hall, 1980.

Kotter, John P. *Organizational Dynamics: Diagnosis and Intervention.* Reading, Mass.: Addison-Wesley Publishing, 1978.

Kotter, John P., and Lawrence, Paul R. *Mayors In Action.* New York: John Wiley & Sons, 1974.

Lawrence, Paul R., and Davis, Dyer. *Renewing American Industry.* New York: Free Press, 1983.

Levitt, Theodore. *Marketing for Business Growth.* New York: McGraw-Hill, 1969.

_____. *Innovation in Marketing: New Perspectives for Profit and Growth.* New York: McGraw-Hill, 1962.

McCarthy, E. Jerome. *Basic Marketing: A Managerial Approach.* 6th ed. Homewood Ill.: Richard D. Irwin, 1978.

Ouchi, William G. *Theory Z: How American Business Can Meet the Japanese Challange.* New York: Avon Books, 1981.

Pascale, Richard T., and Athos, Anthony G. *The Art of Japanese Management.* New York: Simon & Schuster, 1981.

Peters, Thomas J., and Waterman, Robert H., Jr. *The Search of Excellence.* New York: Harper & Row, 1982.

Pfeffer, Jeffrey, and Salancik, Gerald R. *The External Control of Organizations: A Resource Dependence Perspective.* New York: Harper & Row, 1978.

Porter, Michael E. *Competitive Strategy: Techniques for Analyzing Industries and Competitors.* New York: Free Press, 1980.

Quinn, James B. *Strategies for Change: Logical Incrementalism.* Homewood, Ill.: Richard D. Irwin, 1980.

Reader, W. J. *Professional Men.* New York: Basic Books, 1966.

Rhenman, Eric. *Organization Theory for Long-Range Planning.* London, John Wiley & Sons, 1973.

Sacks, Oliver. *Awakenings.* New York: E. P. Dutton, 1983.

Sheldon, Alan. *Managing Change and Collaboration in the Health Field.* Cambridge, Mass.: Oelgeschlager, Gunn and Hain, 1979.

Starr, Paul, *The Social Transformation of American Medicine.* New York: Basic Books, 1982.

Steiner, George A. *Strategic Planning: What Every Manager Must Know.* New York: Free Press, 1979.

————. *Top Management Planning.* London: Macmillan, 1969.

Stonich, P., ed., *Implementing Strategy: Making Strategy Happen.* New York: Ballinger Publishing, 1982.

INDEX